Clinical Heart Failure Management

PRACTICAL RECOMMENDATIONS FOR IMPLEMENTATION

WILLIAM T ABRAHAM | JOHN GF CLELAND
ANDREW JS COATS | EWA JANKOWSKA
MITJA LAINSCAK | YURI LOPATIN | MARCO METRA
GIUSEPPE MC ROSANO | PETAR SEFEROVIC

Otmoor Publishing
for
Radcliffe Cardiology

Otmoor Publishing Ltd for Radcliffe Cardiology
Oxford OX5 2RD
United Kingdom

Barcaray International
Publishing

ISBN-13 978 1 910303 09 2

Typeset and designed by Darkriver Design, Auckland, New Zealand
Cover design by Cox Design, Witney, Oxfordshire, UK

Contents

Preface

Heart failure is a growing epidemic and one of the leading causes of hospitalisations and death throughout the world. Because of its prevalence and associated mortality and morbidity, there has been, throughout the years, the need to better identify the different forms of the disease to gain a better understanding of the underlying mechanisms and the interplay with the different co-morbidities in order to better direct treatments.

The increasing incidence and prevalence of chronic heart failure and our improving ability to identify its main pathophysiological mechanisms has been paralleled by remarkable improvements in medical and device therapy. The developments of new pharmacological and device therapies that have improved the prognosis of patients require a constant update on the overall management strategies of patients with heart failure. International guidelines for the diagnosis and management of heart failure have been recently updated with the most comprehensive and clinically oriented ones, the 2016 ESC/HFA guidelines for the diagnosis and treatment of acute and chronic heart failure, just recently released.

This book covers the recent advances in the diagnosis and the management of this rapidly growing cardiovascular subspecialty and provides an update on guideline-based management of heart failure. Edited by renowned international experts, it is the most updated text on heart failure and a central resource for clinicians caring for patients with heart failure. It offers practical guidance that goes beyond the dry tables of the official guidelines and describes the background, the uncertainties and the newer treatments on the verge of practical implementation.

Device therapies for heart failure with and without mechanical dyssynchrony are constantly in development and most of them have led to a significant improvement in the prognosis of patients with heart failure. This book provides basic knowledge about the modern device management of chronic heart failure and its guideline-based indications. The book also covers practical aspects of the management of patients with heart failure and provides a detailed resource for cardiologists and clinicians. With a strong focus on the medical management of chronic heart failure makes it is a key tool for optimally managing patients with complex co-morbidities.

List of editors and affiliations

William T Abraham
Director of the Division of Cardiovascular Medicine
Professor of Internal Medicine, Physiology and Cell Biology
The Ohio State University Wexner Medical Center.
Columbus, Ohio 43210-1252
United States of America

John GF Cleland
Professor of Clinical Cardiology
National Heart & Lung Institute
Royal Brompton & Harefield Hospitals NHS Trust
Imperial College, London,
United Kingdom

Andrew JS Coats
Joint Academic Vice-President
University of Warwick
UK
and Monash University
Australia

Ewa Jankowska
Professor and Head of Laboratory of Applied Research on Cardiovascular System
Department of Heart Diseases
Wroclaw Medical University, Wroclaw
Poland

Mitja Lainscak
Head of the Research and Education Department
Department of Research and Education
General Hospital Celje
Slovenia

Yuri Lopatin
Professor and Head of Cardiology Department
Volgograd Regional Cardiology Centre, Volgograd
Russia

Marco Metra
Professor of Cardiology
Department of Medical and Surgical Specialties, Radiological Sciences, and Public Health, University of Brescia
Spedali Civili, Brescia
Italy

Giuseppe MC Rosano
Professor of Pharmacology
Consultant Cardiologist
Clinical Academic Group
St George's Hospital NHS Trust
London, United Kingdom
and Scientific Director,
Nutramed Consortium
IRCCS San Raffaele, Roma
Italy

Petar Seferovic
Professor of Internal Medicine – Cardiology
Deputy Director of the Polyclinic of the Clinical Centre of Serbia
Belgrade University School of Medicine, Belgrade
Serbia

1

Definition and classification of heart failure

Introduction

Heart failure is defined by the European Society of Cardiology (ESC) as a clinical syndrome characterised by symptoms such as shortness of breath, persistent coughing or wheezing, ankle swelling and fatigue, that may be accompanied by the following signs: jugular venous pressure, pulmonary crackles, increased heart rate and peripheral oedema.[1] However, these signs may not be present in the early stages and in patients treated with diuretics. When apparent, they are due to a structural and/or functional cardiac abnormality, leading to systolic and/or diastolic ventricular dysfunction, resulting in a reduced cardiac output and/or elevated intra-cardiac pressures at rest or during stress.[2,3] According to the most recent ESC guidelines[1] the initial evaluation of patients with suspected heart failure should include a clinical history and physical examination, laboratory assessment, chest radiography, and electrocardiography. Echocardiography can confirm the diagnosis. Beyond detecting myocardial abnormality, other impairments such as abnormalities of the valves, pericardium, endocardium, heart rhythm, and conduction may be found.[4,2] The identification of the underlying aetiology is pivotal for the diagnosis of heart failure and its treatment.[5]

Clinical course of heart failure

According to the "progressive model",[4] heart failure may be considered as a progressive disorder that starts from a trigger, or "index event", that damages the heart muscle and consequently impairs cardiac myocytes, therefore reducing the myocardium's ability to fill with or eject blood, and finally precluding the heart from contracting normally. This inciting event may have a sudden onset (e.g. myocardial infarction) or a gradual or insidious onset (e.g. haemodynamic pressure or volume overloading), or it may be hereditary. Regardless of the aetiology, the consequence is a decline in pump function of the heart.[4] Also, a progressive, albeit non-linear, decline in health-related quality of life is observed;[6] this course can be interrupted at any time either by sudden cardiac death usually caused by an arrhythmia or can end in a more gradual death caused by progressive pump failure. Patients may also experience progressive episodes of acute decompensation, further reducing the heart's ability to fill with or eject blood appropriately.

Acute heart failure is defined as the rapid onset of symptoms and signs secondary to abnormal cardiac function, which may occur with or without previous cardiac disease.[7] The cardiac dysfunction can be related to systolic or diastolic dysfunction, to abnormalities in cardiac rhythm, or to preload and afterload mismatch.[8] Acute heart failure is often life threatening and requires urgent treatment. In addition, the patient with acute heart failure may present with one of several distinct clinical conditions.[9]

Finally, subclinical forms of heart failure also exist, with asymptomatic cardiac abnormalities. These silent forms of heart failure are considered as its precursors, and should be identified as early intervention may improve outcomes and reduce mortality.[10,11] Unfortunately, subclinical forms of heart failure remain unnoticed and are frequently underdiagnosed.[12] For these reasons, given the heterogeneity of heart failure phenotypes,[13] classification systems and diagnostic algorithms have been developed.

Classifications of heart failure

Heart failure with preserved (HFpEF), mid-range (HFmrEF) and reduced ejection fraction (HFrEF)

From the '90s clinical trials began to select patients based on left ventricular ejection fraction (LVEF), usually measured using echocardiography, a radionuclide technique, or cardiac magnetic resonance. Table 1.1 shows the diagnostic criteria to define heart failure with preserved (HFpEF), mid-range (HFmrEF) and reduced ejection fraction (HFrEF) according to ESC guidelines.[1] Figure 1.1 shows typical echocardiographic pictures of HFrEF and HFpEF.

An old definition for HFpEF was "diastolic' heart failure", as opposed to "systolic" heart failure that corresponded to HFrEF. However, the term diastolic heart failure was replaced by HFpEF given that diastolic dysfunction of

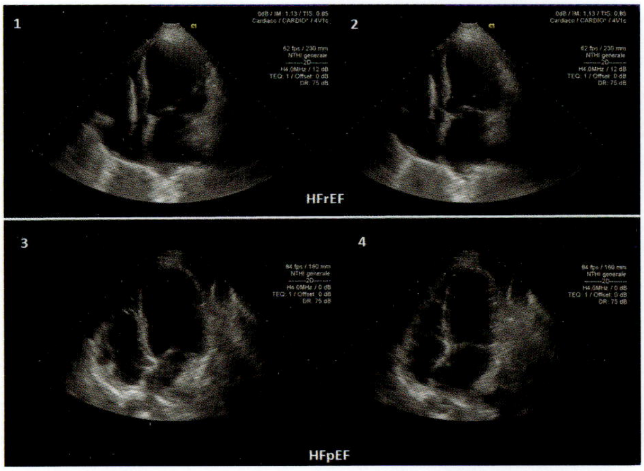

FIGURE 1.1 Echocardiographic differences between heart failure with reduced ejection fraction (HFrEF) and heart failure with preserved ejection fraction (HFpEF) The figure shows echocardiographic images from a patient with HFrEF (above, images 1 and 2) and a patient with HFpEF (below, images 3 and 4). In the images above, ejection fraction (EF) is depressed and the end-systolic volume is increased (image 2). In the right heart chambers electrocatheter is also observable (both images 1 and 2). Conversely, it is noticeable that volumes of the left ventricles as well as EF are preserved in HFpEF (images 3 and 4).

the left ventricle may also characterise HFrEF.[14] On the other hand, the term systolic heart failure was substituted by HFrEF given that subtle abnormalities of systolic function may be also found in patients with HFpEF.[15]

The definition of the range of "normality' of LVEF in heart failure has been long debated.[16,17] According to the European Study Group on Diastolic Heart Failure[18] diagnostic criteria for HFpEF were: a) clinical symptoms and signs; b) normal or mildly reduced LV systolic function (LVEF >50% and LVEDVI <97 mL/m^2); c) diastolic dysfunction. In contrast, criteria from the Framingham study[19] were more pragmatic and less dependent on detailed testing and included: a) clinical symptoms and signs, and b) LVEF ≥50% within 72 h of heart failure; whereas assessment of diastolic function was not needed for diagnosis. Recent and more stringent criteria for HFpEF and HFrEF have been proposed by the new ESC guidelines[1] (see Table 1.1).

Selecting patients according to LVEF is relevant as these heart failure syndromes have distinct patterns of underlying aetiologies, demographics, comorbidities and response to therapies.[2,20] Typically, patients with HFpEF are older, more likely female, and present the following co-morbidities more commonly: arterial hypertension, atrial fibrillation, kidney dysfunction, metabolic

TABLE 1.1 Criteria for diagnosis of heart failure with different LVEF impairment according to ESC guidelines

	Clinical symptoms/signs*	LVEF	Additional criteria
HFpEF	Symptoms: breathlessness, persistent coughing or wheezing, ankle swelling, fatigue, lack of appetite or nausea, impaired thinking. Signs: elevated jugular venous pressure, pulmonary crackles, increased heart rate, and peripheral oedema.	≥ 50%	1. Elevated levels of natriuretic peptides (BNP > 35 pg/ml and/or NT-proBNP > 125 pg/ml); 2. At least one criterion between: a. relevant structural heart disease (LVH and/or LAE), b. diastolic dysfunction
HFmrEF	Symptoms: breathlessness, ankle swelling, fatigue etc. Signs: elevated jugular venous pressure, pulmonary crackles, and peripheral oedema.	40–49%	1. Elevated levels of natriuretic peptides (BNP > 35 pg/ml and/or NT-proBNP > 125 pg/ml); 2. At least one criterion between: a. relevant structural heart disease (LVH and/or LAE), b. diastolic dysfunction
HFrEF	Symptoms: breathlessness, ankle swelling, fatigue etc. Signs: elevated jugular venous pressure, pulmonary crackles, and peripheral oedema.	≤40%	No additional criterion is required.

* Signs may not be present in the early stages of heart failure (especially in HFpEF) and in patients treated with diuretics

BNP = B-type natriuretic peptide; HFmrEF = heart failure with mid-range ejection fraction; HFpEF = heart failure with preserved ejection fraction; HFrEF = heart failure with reduced ejection fraction; LAE = left atrial enlargement; LV = left ventricle; LVEF = left ventricular ejection fraction; LVH = left ventricular hypertrophy; NT-proBNP = N-terminal pro-B type natriuretic peptide.

syndrome, obesity, physical deconditioning, pulmonary disease, pulmonary hypertension and sleep apnoea.[1] Due to polymorbidity, the diagnosis may be more difficult, especially in older adults.[21]

In HFrEF, LVEF is considered as 40% or below. The heart muscle does not contract effectively and less oxygen-rich blood is pumped out to the body. In HFrEF only, therapies have been shown to reduce both morbidity and mortality.[1]

The recent ESC guidelines[1] have finally provided diagnostic criteria for a newly defined group HFmrEF standing for Heart Failure with mid-range Ejection Fraction. Such an 'intermediate group' or 'grey area' presents as mild systolic dysfunction, with a LVEF in the range of 40–49%. Further studies are warranted to clarify its risk factors, demographics, co-morbidities and pathophysiological processes and, consequently, whether its treatments should be similar to those used for HFrEF.[23]

Classifications of heart failure according to the severity of symptoms

The ACC/AHA guidelines have proposed a staging of severity of heart failure based on the structure and damage of the heart muscle.[3] According to this classification, patients may be classified as follows: *Stage A* patients are at high risk for developing heart failure but do not present any structural or functional abnormality or symptoms of heart failure; *Stage B* comprises patients with structural heart disease that is associated with the development of heart failure but signs or symptoms of heart failure are not apparent; *Stage C* includes patients with symptomatic heart failure associated with underlying structural heart disease; *Stage D* patients have advanced structural heart disease and marked symptoms of heart failure at rest despite maximal medical therapy.

A widely-used classification is the New York Heart Association (NYHA) functional classification (1994), which describes heart failure according to severity of its symptoms and impairment of physical activity. *Class I* patients present no limitation in physical activity; therefore symptoms such as breathlessness, fatigue or palpitations are absent during ordinary physical activity. *Class II* includes patients characterised by slight limitation of physical activity. Undue breathlessness, fatigue or palpitations are present during ordinary physical activity, whereas the patient is comfortable at rest. *Class III* comprises patients with a marked limitation of physical activity. The patient is still comfortable at rest, but less than ordinary physical activity results in undue breathlessness, fatigue or palpitations. *Class IV* patients are unable to carry on any physical activity without discomfort and symptoms at rest can also appear.[24] Other classifications developed in the '70s describe the severity of heart failure in the context of acute myocardial infarction, the Killip (1967)[25] and Forrester (1977)[26] classifications.

Advanced heart failure

Advanced heart failure was first defined in 1998 as a syndrome requiring a resting left ventricular ejection fraction <30% and NYHA class III to IV or a peak oxygen uptake (VO_2) below 14 mL/kg/min.[27] In 2004, a U.S. consensus statement defined advanced heart failure as a "state in which patients have significant cardiac dysfunction with marked symptoms of dyspnoea, fatigue,

TABLE 1.2 Advanced heart failure definitions/classifications

HFA position statement 2007 criteria	ESC definition of advanced heart failure in ACCF/AHA 2013 guidelines	INTERMACS classification system
1. Severe symptoms of HF (NYHA class III or IV)	1. Severe symptoms of HF with dyspnoea and/or fatigue at rest or with minima exertion (NYHA class III or IV)	1. Critical cardiogenic shock despite escalating support ("Crash and burn")
2. Episodes of fluid retention and/ or peripheral hypoperfusion	2. Episodes of fluid retention (pulmonary and/or systemic congestion, peripheral edema) and/or reduced cardiac output at rest (peripheral hypoperfusion)	2. Progressive decline with inotrope dependence ("Sliding on inotropes")
3. Objective evidence of severe cardiac dysfunction	3. Objective evidence of severe cardiac dysfunction shown by at least 1 of the following: a. LVEF <30% b. Pseudonormal or restrictive mitral inflow pattern c. Mean PCWP >16 mm HG and/or RAP >12 mm HG by PA catheterisation d. High BNP or NT-proBNP plasma levels in the absence of non-cardiac causes	3. Clinically stable with mild to moderate inotrope dependence ("Dependent stability")
4. Severe impairment of functional capacity	4. Severe impairment of functional capacity shown by one of the following: a. Inability to exercise b. 6-minute walk distance ≤300 m c. Peak VO_2 <12 to 14 IM/kg/min	4. Recurrent, not refractory, advanced HF that can be stabilised ("Frequent flyer")
5. History of ≥1 HF hospitalisation in the past 6 months	5. History of ≥1 HF hospitalisation in past 6 months	5. Exertion intolerant but is comfortable at rest and able to perform activities of daily living with slight difficulty ("Housebound")

HFA position statement 2007 criteria	ESC definition of advanced heart failure in ACCF/AHA 2013 guidelines	INTERMACS classification system
6. Presence of all the previous features despite "attempts to optimise" therapy	6. Presence of all the previous features despite "attempts to optimise" therapy, including diuretics and GDMT, unless these are poorly tolerated or contraindicated, and CRT when indicated	6. Exertion limited; is able to perform mild activity, but fatigue results within a few minutes of any meaningful physical exertion ("Walking wounded")
		7. Advanced NYHA functional class III ("Placeholder")

BNP = B-type natriuretic peptide; CRT = cardiac resynchronization therapy; GDMT = guideline-directed medical therapy; HF = heart failure; INTERMACS = Interagency Registry for Mechanically Assisted Circulatory Support; LVEF = left ventricular ejection fraction; NT-proBNP = N-terminal pro-B type natriuretic peptide; NYHA = New York Heart Association; PA = pulmonary artery; PCWP = pulmonary capillary wedge pressure; RAP = right atrial pressure; VO_2 = oxygen consumption.

or symptoms relating to end-organ hypoperfusion at rest or with minimal exertion despite maximal medical therapy".[28] This definition did not include the criterion of a previous hospitalisation and did not try objectively to assess the impairment of cardiac dysfunction and functional capacity. In 2007, the Heart Failure Association (HFA) of the ESC[9] published a position statement in which the definition and clinical characteristics of advanced chronic heart failure were outlined. According to this definition, both symptoms of severe heart failure and objective evidence of severe cardiac dysfunction, impaired exercise capacity and an unstable clinical course must be present, despite optimal medical treatment. Clinical characteristics and classifications of advanced heart failure are shown in Table 1.2.

The HFA criteria of the ESC were inserted into the AHA/ACC Foundation criteria for destination therapy with cardiac devices.[29] The AHA/ACC guidelines also described heart failure as a progressive disease into four stages from A to D, with stage D being defined as end-stage or advanced heart failure.

The Interagency Registry for Mechanically Assisted Circulatory Support (INTERMACS), a prospective registry that collects data on all patients who receive a durable, FDA approved mechanical circulatory support device in the United States, developed seven profiles that can be used further to stratify patients with advanced heart failure.[30] INTERMACS patient profiles were defined based on clinical descriptors at the time of mechanical circulatory support implant (1=critical cardiogenic shock to 7=advanced NYHA Class III symptoms) (Table 1.2). Such a system classification may be useful to predict outcomes after mechanical assist device implantation.[31]

Despite these classification systems, mostly descriptive, it is vital to realise that a consensus definition for advanced heart failure still needs to be developed. Indeed, there is still considerable variation in the definition of advanced heart failure utilised for clinical trial purposes.[32] Clinicians must recognise the transition to advanced heart failure in order to provide timely and appropriate therapeutic options.[33]

Other definitions of heart failure

End-stage heart failure

Advanced heart failure should be kept distinct from end-stage heart failure. This term indicates an extremely advanced condition where no improvement with conventional heart failure treatment is possible and where palliative care, ventricular assist devices or heart transplantation are indicated. Indeed, there are remarkable differences between advanced and end-stage heart failure in terms of quality of life and outcomes. End-stage heart failure should be also distinguished from acute heart failure in which a certain degree of reversibility can be achieved.[6]

Refractory heart failure

Refractory heart failure is similar to end-stage heart failure and is observed in clinical practice when patients continue to be symptomatic at rest or develop recurrence of heart failure despite optimal contemporary pharmacotherapy proven to be of benefit in clinical trials. Physical examination, laboratory testing, multi-modality imaging, and cardiopulmonary exercise testing are pivotal for the definition of refractory heart failure. These patients commonly have rapid clinical deterioration and may require inotropic agents to augment cardiac performance.[34,35]

References

1. Ponikowski P, Voors AA, Anker SD, Bueno H, Cleland JG, Coats AJ, Falk V, González-Juanatey JR, Harjola VP, Jankowska EA, Jessup M, Linde C, Nihoyannopoulos P, Parissis JT, Pieske B, Riley JP, Rosano GM, Ruilope LM, Ruschitzka F, Rutten FH, van der Meer P; Authors/Task Force Members; Document Reviewers. 2016 ESC Guidelines for the diagnosis and treatment of acute and chronic heart failure: The Task Force for the diagnosis and treatment of acute and chronic heart failure of the European Society of Cardiology (ESC) Developed with the special contribution of the Heart Failure Association (HFA) of the ESC. Eur Heart J. 2016 May 20. pii: ehw128. PMID: 27206819.
2. McMurray JJ, Adamopoulos S, Anker SD et al. ESC Guidelines for the diagnosis and treatment of acute and chronic heart failure 2012: The Task Force for the Diagnosis and Treatment of Acute and Chronic Heart Failure 2012 of the European Society of Cardiology. Developed in collaboration with the Heart Failure Association (HFA) of the ESC. Eur Heart J. 2012; 33: 1787–1847.
3. Hunt SA, Abraham WT, Chin MH et al. 2009 focused update incorporated into the ACC/AHA 2005 guidelines for the diagnosis and management of heart failure in adults: a report of the American College of Cardiology Foundation/American Heart Association Task Force on Practice Guidelines: developed in collaboration with the International Society for Heart and Lung Transplantation. Circulation. 2009; 119(14): e391–e479.
4. Mann DL, Bristow MR. Mechanisms and models in heart failure: the biomechanical model and beyond. Circulation. 2005 May 31; 111(21): 2837–2849.
5. King M, Kingery J, Casey B. Diagnosis and Evaluation of Heart Failure. Am Fam Physician. 2012 Jun 15; 85(12): 1161–1168.
6. Metra M, Ponikowski P, Dickstein K et al. Advanced chronic heart failure: A position statement from the Study Group on Advanced Heart Failure of the Heart Failure Association of the European Society of Cardiology. Eur J Heart Fail. 2007; 9: 684–94.
7. Gheorghiade M, Zannad F, Sopko G et al. Acute heart failure syndromes: current state and framework for future research. Circulation. 2005 Dec 20; 112(25): 3958–68.
8. Dickstein K, Cohen-Solal A, Filippatos G et al. ESC guidelines for the diagnosis and treatment of acute and chronic heart failure 2008: the Task Force for the diagnosis and treatment of acute and chronic heart failure 2008 of the European Society of Cardiology. Developed in collaboration with the Heart Failure Association of the ESC (HFA) and endorsed by the European Society of Intensive Care Medicine (ESICM). Eur J Heart Fail. 2008 Oct; 10(10): 933–89. doi:10.1016/j.ejheart.2008.08.005. Epub 2008 Sep 16. Review. Erratum in: Eur J Heart Fail. 2009 Jan; 11(1): 110. Eur J Heart Fail. 2010 Apr; 12(4): 416. Dosage error in article text. PMID: 18826876.
9. Nieminen MS, Bohm M, Cowie MR et al. Executive summary of the guidelines on the diagnosis and treatment of acute heart failure: the Task Force on Acute Heart Failure of the European Society of Cardiology. Eur Heart J. 2005; 26: 384–416.
10. Wang TJ. Natural history of asymptomatic left ventricular systolic dysfunction in the 3746 community. Circulation. 2003; 108: 977–982. 3747.
11. The SOLVD Investigators. Effect of enalapril on mortality and the development of heart

3748 failure in asymptomatic patients with reduced left ventricular ejection fractions. N Engl J 3749 Med. 1992; 327: 685–691.
12. Schocken DD, Benjamin EJ, Fonarow GC et al. Prevention of heart failure: a scientific statement from the American Heart Association Councils on Epidemiology and Prevention, Clinical Cardiology, Cardiovascular Nursing, and High Blood Pressure Research; Quality of Care and Outcomes Research Interdisciplinary Working Group; and Functional Genomics and Translational Biology Interdisciplinary Working Group. Circulation. 2008; 117: 2544–2565.
13. Senni M, Paulus WJ, Gavazzi A et al. New strategies for heart failure with preserved ejection fraction: the importance of targeted therapies for heart failure phenotypes. Eur Heart J. 2014 Oct 21; 35(40): 2797–815. doi:10.1093/eurheartj/ehu204.
14. Borlaug B, Paulus W. Heart failure with preserved ejection fraction: pathophysiology, diagnosis, and treatment Eur Heart J. 2011 Mar; 32(6): 670–679.
15. Shah AM, Claggett B, Sweitzer NK et al. Prognostic Importance of Impaired Systolic Function in Heart Failure With Preserved Ejection Fraction and the Impact of Spironolactone. Circulation. 2015 Aug 4; 132(5): 402–14. doi:10.1161/CIRCULATIONAHA.115.015884.
16. Davies M, Hobbs F, Davis R et al. Prevalence of left-ventricular systolic dysfunction and heart failure in the Echocardiographic Heart of England Screening study: a population based study. Lancet. 2001 Aug 11; 358(9280): 439–44.
17. Petrie M, McMurray J. Changes in notions about heart failure. Lancet. 2001 Aug 11; 58(9280): 432–4.
18. Paulus WJ, Tschope C, Sanderson JE et al. How to diagnose diastolic heart failure: a consensus statement on the diagnosis of heart failure with normal left ventricular ejection fraction by the Heart Failure and Echocardiography Associations of the European Society of Cardiology. Eur Heart J. 2007; 28: 2539–2550.
19. Vasan RS, Levy D. Defining diastolic heart failure: a call for standardized diagnostic criteria. Circulation. 2000; 101: 2118–2121.
20. Butler J, Fonarow GC, Zile MR et al. Developing therapies for heart failure with preserved ejection fraction: current state and future directions. JACC Heart Fail. 2014; 2: 97–3756 112.
21. Bhuiyan T, Maurer MS. Heart Failure with Preserved Ejection Fraction: Persistent Diagnosis, Therapeutic Enigma. Curr Cardiovasc Risk Rep. 2011 Oct; 5(5): 440–449.
22. Iwano, William C. Little Shah SJ, Katz DH, Deo RC. Phenotypic Spectrum of Heart Failure with Preserved Ejection Fraction. Heart Fail Clin. 2014 July; 10(3): 407–418.
23. Lam CSP, Solomon SD. The middle child in heart failure: heart failure with mid-range ejection fraction (40–50%). Eur J Heart Fail. 2014; 16: 1049–1055.
24. The Criteria Committee of the New York Heart Association. Nomenclature and Criteria for Diagnosis of Diseases of the Heart and Great Vessels. 9th ed. Little Brown & Co; 1994. pp 253–256.
25. Killip T, 3rd, Kimball JT. Treatment of myocardial infarction in a coronary care unit. A two year experience with 250 patients. Am J Cardiol. 1967; 20: 457–464.
26. Forrester JS, Diamond GA, Swan HJ. Correlative classification of clinical and hemodynamic function after acute myocardial infarction. Am J Cardiol. 1977; 39: 137–145.

27. Adams KF, Jr., Zannad F. Clinical definition and epidemiology of advanced heart failure. Am Heart J. 1998; 135:S204–15.
28. Goodlin SJ, Hauptman PJ, Arnold R et al. Consensus statement: palliative and supportive care in advanced heart failure. J Card Fail. 2004; 10: 200–9.
29. Yancy CW, Jessup M, Bozkurt B et al. 2013 ACCF/AHA Guideline for the Management of Heart Failure: A Report of the American College of Cardiology Foundation/American Heart Association Task Force on Practice Guidelines. J Am Coll Cardiol. 2013; 62: e147–239.
30. Stevenson LW, Pagani FD, Young JB, Jessup M, Miller L, Kormos RL, Naftel DC, Ulisney K, Desvigne-Nickens P, Kirklin JK. INTERMACS profiles of advanced heart failure: the current picture. J Heart Lung Transplant. 2009 Jun; 28(6): 535–41.
31. Alba AC, Rao V, Ivanov J, Ross HJ, Delgado DH. Usefulness of the INTERMACS scale to predict outcomes after mechanical assist device implantation. J Heart Lung Transplant. 2009: 827–33.
32. Bjork JB, Alton KK, Georgiopoulou VV, Butler J, Kalogeropoulos AP. Defining Advanced Heart Failure: A Systematic Review of Criteria Used in Clinical Trials, Journal of Cardiac Failure (2016), http://dx.doi.org/doi:10.1016/j.cardfail.2016.03.003.
33. Allen LA, Stevenson LW, Grady KL et al. Decision making in advanced heart failure: a scientific statement from the American Heart Association. Circulation. 2012; 125: 1928–1952.
34. Hunt SA, Abraham WT, Chin MH et al. ACC/AHA 2005 guideline update for the diagnosis and management of chronic heart failure in the adult-summary article. A report of the American College of Cardiology/American Heart Association. Task Force on Practice Guidelines (Writing Committee to Update the 2001 Guidelines for the Evaluation and Management of Heart Failure). J Am Coll Cardiol. 2005; 46: 1116–1143.
35. Ahmad T, Patel CB, Milano CA, Rogers JG. When the heart runs out of heartbeats: treatment options for refractory end-stage heart failure. Circulation. 2012; 125: 2948–2955.

2

Epidemiology and prognosis of heart failure

Introduction

In this chapter the state of the art of prevalence, incidence and prognosis of heart failure is discussed. Prevalence and incidence are two measures of disease occurrence. Briefly, prevalence is the proportion of the population affected by the disease at a certain point in time. Incidence indicates the number of new cases within a given time period in a population at risk for the disease (for example, elderly people). A related, prognostic measure is mortality, i.e. the incidence of death from the disease occurring in a period of time. In the case of chronic, steady-state disease such as heart failure, disease duration is directly affected by mortality, and prevalence may correspond to the incidence of disease multiplied by the average duration of disease.[1] Prevalence rates of heart failure may, therefore, vary across studies depending on the variability in incidence as well as in survival between population samples.[1] Also, given that heart failure is a complex syndrome with different phenotypes (see Chapter 1), each with specific clinical characteristics and associated risk factors, prevalence and incidence rates may vary according to the definition of the heart failure subtype.[2] Finally, rates may vary on the basis of the method of collecting data and the criterion for defining left ventricular systolic dysfunction that is applied in the study.[3]

Prevalence and incidence of heart failure

Heart failure represents an increasing issue for global healthcare systems. Even before the millenium a prevalence of 23 million individuals living with heart failure is estimated worldwide.[4] However, epidemiological data predominantly derive from North America and Europe[3] with overall prevalence rates of 1–2%.[1] In particular, the current prevalence is up to 3%.[5] Also, the prevalence of heart failure is growing despite substantial improvements in its management, and for this reason heart failure represents an exception among cardiovascular disorders.[6] Indeed, from the 1970s to 1990s, an epidemic was declared,[7] due to a steep rise in prevalence and hospitalisation rates.[8] Since then, the worldwide prevalence of heart failure has progressively increased, although this mainly relates to increases in crude prevalence rates, with standardised rates even decreasing somewhat due to the ageing population and improved survival after acute MI for example.

One of the possible explanations for this growth is that heart failure is predominantly a disease of the elderly. Indeed, its prevalence rises with age, increasing sharply from 1% in 40-year-old individuals, affecting about 10% of men and 8% of women aged more than 60 years, and exceeding 10% in both sexes over the age of 70 years.[9] Indeed, among elderly people (≥65 years) referred to primary care services for shortness of breath on exertion, 1 out of 6 presents with previously unrecognised heart failure, mainly heart failure with preserved ejection fraction (HFpEF).[10,11] Also, more than 80% of the deaths and prevalent cases of heart failure occur among people aged ≥65 years.[1] Other explanations for the growing prevalence of heart failure may be the increasing incidence and, paradoxically, advances in awareness and diagnosis as well as in management.[1] Also this trend mirrors the increasing prevalence of major heart failure risk factors, including obesity and diabetes.[12]

As for prevalence, the incidence of heart failure is greater in males and in the elderly, especially for HFpEF.[1] In the Framingham Heart study[13] conducted from 1950 to 1999, the incidence of heart failure was nearly 5.6 in men and 3.3 in women per 1,000 person-years but remained unchanged in men whilst it decreased in women. In the Olmsted County study[14] the incidence was nearly 3.8 and 2.9 per 1,000 person-years, respectively, and remained stable between 1979 and 2000 in both sexes. Beyond age and gender, further studies have also highlighted epidemiological differences according to the heart failure syndrome (mainly HFpEF and heart failure with reduced ejection fraction (HFrEF)).[15–22] It is now acknowledged that there are pathophysiological characteristics and specific associated risk factors for each heart failure subtype.[2]

Prevalence and incidence of heart failure syndromes

Patients with HFpEF are more often older, female, and with a history of hypertension and atrial fibrillation than those with HFrEF, whilst a history of myocardial infarction is less frequent.[23–24] In a recent European retrospective cohort study,[15] based on admissions in 2012, only 17% of heart failure patients had HFpEF type whilst the 83% were diagnosed with HFrEF. However, there is inconsistency across studies for the prevalence rates of HFpEF, generally ranging from 22% to 73%.[25–32,24,11] Such variability probably depends on the definition of HFpEF (e.g. what is the 'normality' threshold of ejection fraction) and, consequently, sample inclusion criteria.[33] Also the clinical setting (e.g. primary care, hospital clinic, etc.) plays a role in determining the differences of prevalence across studies. Other characteristics of the study samples affecting prevalence rates are age, gender and history of myocardial infarction.[2]

Heterogeneous data also exist with regard to advanced heart failure, whose prevalence ranges from 1 to 10% of the total heart failure population.[34] As for HFpEF, this variability probably depends on the application of different definitions of this syndrome and epidemiological criteria across studies.[35]

As for incidence, a substudy of the Prevention of Renal and Vascular End-stage Disease (PREVEND),[36] a European community-based cohort study, showed a higher percentage of new cases of HFrEF compared with HFpEF (66 vs. 34%, respectively) than other community-based studies.[33,37] Since patients with HFrEF are more often younger than HFpEF, these incidence rates may presumably be elucidated considering the younger age of this cohort (middle-age). In line with this explanation, there is evidence that incidence of HFrEF is decreasing among hospitalised patients at a greater extent than that of HFpEF.[22,38]

Taking into account the available evidence, more studies are warranted to clarify prevalence and incidence rates of HFrEF. In fact, a much greater wealth of epidemiological data on HFpEF has been collected so far. Moreover, heart failure with mid-range ejection fraction (HFmrEF) has been completely neglected by epidemiological studies, as these patients –who stand in a "grey area" (see Chapter 1) are usually excluded from study selection criteria. After the recent standard definition of HFmrEF from the European guidelines,[2] upcoming epidemiological research will hopefully include patients with this syndrome to clarify its prevalence, incidence and prognostic correlates.

Prognosis of heart failure

Heart failure is associated with a poor long-term prognosis. Nearly 50% of patients with this diagnosis die within 4 years.[12] Also, heart failure leads to impairment in quality of life due to its very disabling symptoms.[39] Heart failure is still the most common cause of hospitalisation in industrialised countries. A study from the European Society of Cardiology[40] reported a 12-month hospitalisation rate of 44% and a mortality rate for any cause of 17% in hospitalised

TABLE 2.1 Markers of worse prognosis

Socio-demographic characteristics	Older age, male sex, low socioeconomic status
Clinical markers	Severity of heart failure, myocardial remodeling and severity of heart dysfunction
Biomarkers	Markers of neurohormonal activation, markers of renal function, markers of inflammation, markers of cardiac damage/dysfunction, and other markers. Specific genetic mutations
Cardiovascular comorbidities	Atrial fibrillation, ventricular arrhythmia, non-revascularizable coronary artery disease, previous stroke/TIA, peripheral arterial disease
Non-cardiovascular comorbidities	Diabetes, anaemia, iron deficiency, chronic obstructive pulmonary disease, renal failure, liver dysfunction, sleep apnoea, cognitive impairment and depression
Others	Non-adherence with treatment, heart failure hospitalisation, aborted cardiac arrest, implantable cardioverter-defibrillator shock

Adapted from: reference 2.

patients; and 32% and 7% respectively in stable/ambulatory patients. In this study, sudden death and worsening heart failure were the most common modes of death for the patients.

Despite the fact that all-cause mortality is reported in some studies to be higher in HFrEF than HFpEF,[40–42] both the syndromes carry a similarly poor prognosis[15] and their hospitalisation rates are comparable.[15,20,43–45] Overall, annual hospital discharges associated with heart failure are decreasing in Europe, and a consequent slight improvement in survival is observed in heart failure patients.[46–47] Such an improvement in survival has been observed in both men and women,[13,48] and along with the ageing of the population can presumably lead to a steep rise in prevalence in spite of stable incidence rates.[33] Also, there is a change in the distribution of the causes of death (and also hospitalisation) toward non-cardiovascular causes in heart failure patients, consistent with the increased occurrence of non-cardiovascular comorbidities.[48] This trend toward non-cardiovascular causes of death is more evident for HFpEF[14] and is suggestive of the key role of comorbidities in heart failure, particularly the HFpEF pattern.[49]

Thus, despite the encouraging European data on survival, the outcome is still poor.[2] For this reason, markers of worse prognosis have been identified to help clinicians (Table 2.1). Unfortunately, their clinical applicability is still limited[2] and, therefore, more studies are warranted.

In summary, survival after the diagnosis of heart failure remains unsatisfactory but has improved substantially over time. This trend, along with the aforementioned trend in incidence, indicates that heart failure is "an epidemic of hospitalizations among survivors who now live longer with the disease".[48]

References

1. Bui, A. L., T. B. Horwich and G. C. Fonarow (2011). Epidemiology and risk profile of heart failure. Nat Rev Cardiol 8(1): 30–41.
2. Ponikowski P, Voors AA, Anker SD, Bueno H, Cleland JG, Coats AJ, Falk V, González-Juanatey JR, Harjola VP, Jankowska EA, Jessup M, Linde C, Nihoyannopoulos P, Parissis JT, Pieske B, Riley JP, Rosano GM, Ruilope LM, Ruschitzka F, Rutten FH, van der Meer P; Authors/Task Force Members; Document Reviewers. 2016 ESC Guidelines for the diagnosis and treatment of acute and chronic heart failure. Eur J Heart Fail. 2016 May 20. doi:10.1002/ejhf.592.
3. Guha, K. and T. McDonagh (2013). Heart failure epidemiology: European perspective. Curr Cardiol Rev 9(2): 123–127.
4. McMurray, J. J., M. C. Petrie, D. R. Murdoch and A. P. Davie (1998). Clinical epidemiology of heart failure: public and private health burden. Eur Heart J. 19 Suppl P: P9–16.
5. van Riet EE, Hoes AW, Wagenaar KP, Limburg A, Landman MA, Rutten FH. Epidemiology of heart failure: the prevalence of heart failure and ventricular dysfunction in older adults over time. A systematic review. Eur J Heart Fail. 2016 Mar; 18(3): 242–52. doi:10.1002/ejhf.483.
6. Braunwald, E. (2013). Heart failure. JACC Heart Fail. 1(1): 1–20.
7. McCullough, P. A., E. F. Philbin, J. A. Spertus, S. Kaatz, K. R. Sandberg, W. D. Weaver and S. Resource Utilization Among Congestive Heart Failure (2002). Confirmation of a heart failure epidemic: findings from the Resource Utilization Among Congestive Heart Failure (REACH) study. J Am Coll Cardiol. 39(1): 60–69.
8. Hoes, A. W., A. Mosterd and D. E. Grobbee. (1998). An epidemic of heart failure? Recent evidence from Europe. Eur Heart J. 19 Suppl L: L2–9.
9. Rich, M. W. (2001). Heart failure in the 21st century: a cardiogeriatric syndrome. J Gerontol A Biol Sci Med Sci. 56(2): M88–96.
10. Filippatos, G. and J. T. Parissis (2011). Heart failure diagnosis and prognosis in the elderly: the proof of the pudding is in the eating. Eur J Heart Fail. 13(5): 467–471.
11. van Riet, E. E., A. W. Hoes, A. Limburg, M. A. Landman, H. van der Hoeven and F. H. Rutten (2014). Prevalence of unrecognized heart failure in older persons with shortness of breath on exertion. Eur J Heart Fail. 16(7): 772–777.
12. Lopez-Sendòn, J. (2011). The heart failure epidemic. Medicographia. 33: 363–369.
13. Levy, D., S. Kenchaiah, M. G. Larson, E. J. Benjamin, M. J. Kupka, K. K. Ho, J. M. Murabito and R. S. Vasan (2002). Long-term trends in the incidence of and survival with heart failure. N Engl J Med. 347(18): 1397–1402.
14. Roger, V. L., S. A. Weston, M. M. Redfield, J. P. Hellermann-Homan, J. Killian, B. P. Yawn and S. J. Jacobsen (2004). Trends in heart failure incidence and survival in a community-based population. JAMA. 292(3): 344–350.

15. Dulai, R., A. S. Sheikh, A. Qureshi, S. Katechia, Y. Peysakhova, M. Johns and S. Mazhar (2016). Prevalence, clinical characteristics and outcomes of HF with preserved versus reduced ejection fraction. Br J Cardiol. 23(1).
16. Lee, D. S., P. Gona, R. S. Vasan, M. G. Larson, E. J. Benjamin, T. J. Wang, J. V. Tu and D. Levy (2009). Relation of disease pathogenesis and risk factors to heart failure with preserved or reduced ejection fraction: insights from the framingham heart study of the national heart, lung, and blood institute. Circulation. 119(24): 3070–3077.
17. Fonarow, G. C., W. G. Stough, W. T. Abraham, N. M. Albert, M. Gheorghiade, B. H. Greenberg, C. M. O'Connor, J. L. Sun, C. W. Yancy, J. B. Young, O.-H. Investigators and Hospitals (2007). Characteristics, treatments, and outcomes of patients with preserved systolic function hospitalized for heart failure: a report from the OPTIMIZE-HF Registry. J Am Coll Cardiol. 50(8): 768–777.
18. Yancy, C. W., M. Lopatin, L. W. Stevenson, T. De Marco, G. C. Fonarow, A. S. A. Committee and Investigators (2006). Clinical presentation, management, and in-hospital outcomes of patients admitted with acute decompensated heart failure with preserved systolic function: a report from the Acute Decompensated Heart Failure National Registry (ADHERE) Database. J Am Coll Cardiol. 47(1): 76–84.
19. Vasan, R. S., E. J. Benjamin and D. Levy (1995). Prevalence, clinical features and prognosis of diastolic heart failure: an epidemiologic perspective. J Am Coll Cardiol. 26(7): 1565–1574.
20. Lenzen, M. J., W. J. Scholte op Reimer, E. Boersma, P. J. Vantrimpont, F. Follath, K. Swedberg, J. Cleland and M. Komajda (2004). Differences between patients with a preserved and a depressed left ventricular function: a report from the EuroHeart Failure Survey. Eur Heart J. 25(14): 1214–1220.
21. Bursi, F., S. A. Weston, M. M. Redfield, S. J. Jacobsen, S. Pakhomov, V. T. Nkomo, R. A. Meverden and V. L. Roger (2006). Systolic and diastolic heart failure in the community. JAMA. 296(18): 2209–2216.
22. Owan, T. E., D. O. Hodge, R. M. Herges, S. J. Jacobsen, V. L. Roger and M. M. Redfield (2006). Trends in prevalence and outcome of heart failure with preserved ejection fraction. N Engl J Med. 355(3): 251–259.
23. Bleumink, G. S., A. M. Knetsch, M. C. Sturkenboom, S. M. Straus, A. Hofman, J. W. Deckers, J. C. Witteman and B. H. Stricker (2004). Quantifying the heart failure epidemic: prevalence, incidence rate, lifetime risk and prognosis of heart failure The Rotterdam Study. Eur Heart J. 25(18): 1614–1619.
24. Maggioni AP, Anker SD, Dahlström U, et al. Are hospitalized or ambulatory patients with heart failure treated in accordance with European Society of Cardiology guidelines? Evidence from 12,440 patients of the ESC Heart Failure Long-Term Registry. Eur J Heart Fail. 2013 Oct; 15(10): 1173–84. doi:10.1093/eurjhf/hft134.
25. Ceia, F., C. Fonseca, T. Mota, H. Morais, F. Matias, A. de Sousa, A. Oliveira and E. Investigators (2002). Prevalence of chronic heart failure in Southwestern Europe: the EPICA study. Eur J Heart Fail. 4(4): 531–539.
26. Hellermann, J. P., S. J. Jacobsen, G. S. Reeder, F. Lopez-Jimenez, S. A. Weston and V. L. Roger (2003). Heart failure after myocardial infarction: prevalence of preserved left ventricular systolic function in the community. Am Heart J. 145(4): 742–748.
27. Badano, L. P., M. C. Albanese, P. De Biaggio, P. Rozbowsky, D. Miani, C. Fresco and P.

M. Fioretti (2004). Prevalence, clinical characteristics, quality of life, and prognosis of patients with congestive heart failure and isolated left ventricular diastolic dysfunction. J Am Soc Echocardiogr. 17(3): 253–261.

28. Peyster, E., J. Norman and M. Domanski (2004). Prevalence and predictors of heart failure with preserved systolic function: community hospital admissions of a racially and gender diverse elderly population. J Card Fail. 10(1): 49–54.
29. Boonman-de Winter, L. J., F. H. Rutten, M. J. Cramer, M. J. Landman, A. H. Liem, G. E. Rutten and A. W. Hoes (2012). High prevalence of previously unknown heart failure and left ventricular dysfunction in patients with type 2 diabetes. Diabetologia. 55(8): 2154–2162.
30. Mureddu, G. F., N. Agabiti, V. Rizzello, F. Forastiere, R. Latini, G. Cesaroni, S. Masson, G. Cacciatore, F. Colivicchi, M. Uguccioni, C. A. Perucci, A. Boccanelli and P. S. Group (2012). Prevalence of preclinical and clinical heart failure in the elderly. A population-based study in Central Italy. Eur J Heart Fail. 14(7): 718–729.
31. Tiller, D., M. Russ, K. H. Greiser, S. Nuding, H. Ebelt, A. Kluttig, J. A. Kors, J. Thiery, M. Bruegel, J. Haerting and K. Werdan (2013). Prevalence of symptomatic heart failure with reduced and with normal ejection fraction in an elderly general population-the CARLA study. PLoS One. 8(3): e59225.
32. van Riet, E. E., A. W. Hoes, K. P. Wagenaar, A. Limburg, M. A. Landman and F. H. Rutten (2016). Epidemiology of heart failure: the prevalence of heart failure and ventricular dysfunction in older adults over time. A systematic review. Eur J Heart Fail. 18(3): 242–252.
33. Lam, C. S., E. Donal, E. Kraigher-Krainer and R. S. Vasan (2011). Epidemiology and clinical course of heart failure with preserved ejection fraction. Eur J Heart Fail. 13(1): 18–28.
34. Fang, J. C., G. A. Ewald, L. A. Allen, J. Butler, C. A. Westlake Canary, M. Colvin-Adams, M. G. Dickinson, P. Levy, W. G. Stough, N. K. Sweitzer, J. R. Teerlink, D. J. Whellan, N. M. Albert, R. Krishnamani, M. W. Rich, M. N. Walsh, M. R. Bonnell, P. E. Carson, M. C. Chan, D. L. Dries, A. F. Hernandez, R. E. Hershberger, S. D. Katz, S. Moore, J. E. Rodgers, J. G. Rogers, A. R. Vest, M. M. Givertz and C. Heart Failure Society of America Guidelines (2015). Advanced (stage D) heart failure: a statement from the Heart Failure Society of America Guidelines Committee. J Card Fail. 21(6): 519–534.
35. Bjork, J. B., K. K. Alton, V. V. Georgiopoulou, J. Butler and A. P. Kalogeropoulos (2016). Defining Advanced Heart Failure: A Systematic Review of Criteria Used in Clinical Trials. J Card Fail. 2016 Mar 11. pii: S1071–9164(16)00076-2. doi:0.1016/j.cardfail.2016.03.003. [Epub ahead of print]
36. Brouwers, F. P., R. A. de Boer, P. van der Harst, A. A. Voors, R. T. Gansevoort, S. J. Bakker, H. L. Hillege, D. J. van Veldhuisen and W. H. van Gilst (2013). Incidence and epidemiology of new onset heart failure with preserved vs. reduced ejection fraction in a community-based cohort: 11-year follow-up of PREVEND. Eur Heart J. 34(19): 1424–1431.
37. Ho, J. E., A. Lyass, D. S. Lee, R. S. Vasan, W. B. Kannel, M. G. Larson and D. Levy (2013). Predictors of new-onset heart failure: differences in preserved versus reduced ejection fraction. Circ Heart Fail. 6(2): 279–286.

38. Gerber, Y., S. A. Weston, M. M. Redfield, A. M. Chamberlain, S. M. Manemann, R. Jiang, J. M. Killian and V. L. Roger (2015). A contemporary appraisal of the heart failure epidemic in Olmsted County, Minnesota, 2000 to 2010. JAMA Intern Med. 175(6): 996–1004.
39. Vongmany, J., L. D. Hickman, J. Lewis, P. J. Newton and J. L. Phillips (2016). Anxiety in chronic heart failure and the risk of increased hospitalisations and mortality: A systematic review. Eur J Cardiovasc Nurs. pii: 1474515116635923. [Epub ahead of print]
40. Maggioni, A. P., U. Dahlstrom, G. Filippatos, O. Chioncel, M. Crespo Leiro, J. Drozdz, F. Fruhwald, L. Gullestad, D. Logeart, G. Fabbri, R. Urso, M. Metra, J. Parissis, H. Persson, P. Ponikowski, M. Rauchhaus, A. A. Voors, O. W. Nielsen, F. Zannad, L. Tavazzi and C. Heart Failure Association of the European Society of (2013). EURObservational Research Programme: regional differences and 1-year follow-up results of the Heart Failure Pilot Survey (ESC-HF Pilot). Eur J Heart Fail. 15(7): 808–817.
41. Somaratne, J. B., C. Berry, J. J. McMurray, K. K. Poppe, R. N. Doughty and G. A. Whalley (2009). The prognostic significance of heart failure with preserved left ventricular ejection fraction: a literature-based meta-analysis. Eur J Heart Fail. 11(9): 855–862.
42. Pocock, S. J., C. A. Ariti, J. J. McMurray, A. Maggioni, L. Kober, I. B. Squire, K. Swedberg, J. Dobson, K. K. Poppe, G. A. Whalley, R. N. Doughty and F. Meta-Analysis Global Group in Chronic Heart (2013). Predicting survival in heart failure: a risk score based on 39 372 patients from 30 studies. Eur Heart J. 34(19): 1404–1413.
43. Berry, C., K. Hogg, J. Norrie, K. Stevenson, M. Brett and J. McMurray (2005). Heart failure with preserved left ventricular systolic function: a hospital cohort study. Heart. 91(7): 907–913.
44. Gotsman, I., D. Zwas, D. Planer, T. Azaz-Livshits, D. Admon, C. Lotan and A. Keren (2008). Clinical outcome of patients with heart failure and preserved left ventricular function. Am J Med. 121(11): 997–1001.
45. Gotsman, I., D. Zwas, C. Lotan and A. Keren (2012). Heart failure and preserved left ventricular function: long term clinical outcome. PLoS One. 7(7): e41022.
46. Jhund, P. S., K. Macintyre, C. R. Simpson, J. D. Lewsey, S. Stewart, A. Redpath, J. W. Chalmers, S. Capewell and J. J. McMurray (2009). Long-term trends in first hospitalization for heart failure and subsequent survival between 1986 and 2003: a population study of 5.1 million people. Circulation. 119(4): 515–523.
47. Laribi, S., A. Aouba, M. Nikolaou, J. Lassus, A. Cohen-Solal, P. Plaisance, G. Pavillon, P. Jois, GC. Fonarow, E. Jougla, A. Mebazaa and G. network (2012). Trends in death attributed to heart failure over the past two decades in Europe. Eur J Heart Fail. 14(3): 234–239.
48. Roger, V. L. (2013). Epidemiology of heart failure. Circ Res. 113(6): 646–659.
49. Pardeep S. Jhund and Luigi Tavazzi. Has the 'epidemic' of heart failure been replaced by a tsunami of co-morbidities? Eur J Heart Failure. (2016); in press. doi:10.1002/ejhf.529

3

Clinical diagnosis in heart failure

Introduction

The new ESC guidelines[1] have provided updated evidence-based recommendations for the clinical diagnosis of heart failure. Box 3.1 summarises the diagnostic process in the case of a patient presenting with acute dyspnoea and

BOX 3.1 Diagnostic assessment in patient with acute heart failure adapted from the ESC guidelines (2016)[1]

1. Measurement of plasma natriuretic peptide level (BNP, NT-proBNP or MR-proANP)*
2. a) 12-lead ECG;
   b) chest X-ray†
   c) laboratory assessments: cardiac troponins, BUN (or urea), creatinine, electrolytes (sodium, potassium), glucose, complete blood count, liver function tests and TSH.
3. Echocardiography‡

* to help in the differentiation of acute heart failure from non-cardiac causes of acute dyspnea

† to assess signs of pulmonary congestion and detect other cardiac or non-cardiac diseases that may cause or contribute to the patient's symptoms

‡ recommended immediately in haemodynamically unstable patients with acute heart failure and within 48 hours when cardiac structure and function are either not known or may have changed since previous studies.

suspected acute heart failure. Table 3.1 summarises the diagnostic elements that should be assessed in a patient with non-acute onset, as described below. The diagnostic process is illustrated in an algorithm developed by the ESC with an adaption shown in Figure 3.1.[1]

Initial assessment

In patients with non-acute onset, presenting with symptoms or signs of heart failure non-urgently in primary care or in a hospital outpatient clinic, the probability of heart failure should first be evaluated by assessing history and symptomatology and with physical examination (Table 3.1). During these steps, at least one element should be abnormal to continue to consider a

TABLE 3.1 Diagnostic assessments in patient with suspected heart failure (non acute onset) according to the ESC guidelines (2016)[1]

Clinical history	History of CAD (MI, revascularization) History of arterial hypertension Exposure to cardiotoxic drug/radiation Use of diuretics Orthopnoea/paroxysmal nocturnal dyspnea
Physical examination	Rales Bilateral ankle oedema Heart murmur Jugular venous dilatation Laterally displaced/broadened apical beat
Echocardiography	Myocardial abnormality Abnormalities of the valves, pericardium, endocardium, heart rhythm, or conduction
Laboratory exams	Complete blood count Serum electrolytes Liver function tests Renal function tests Serum glucose Thyroid-stimulating hormone Urinalysis Troponin Natriuretic peptides Arterial blood gases

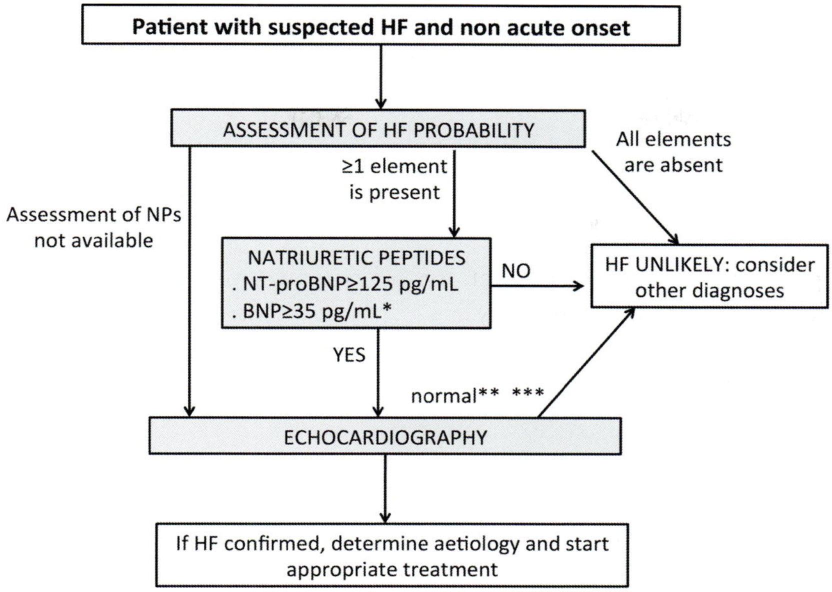

FIGURE 3.1 Algorithm for the diagnosis of heart failure in non-acute setting.
HF = heart failure; NPs = plasma natriuretic peptides
*not suitable for patients taking angiotensin receptor neprilysin inhibitors
** normal ventricular and atrial volumes and function
***consider other causes of elevated natriuretic peptides

diagnostic hypothesis of heart failure (Figure 3.1). If so, plasma natriuretic peptides (NPs) should be measured. This measurement will allow informed decision-making as to whether the patient needs to undergo an echocardiogram (see paragraph below). If no abnormalities are found, heart failure is unlikely and other diagnoses should be considered. Echocardiography is also a first-step option, e.g. if more available or if it is deemed that the diagnostic yield would be higher.

Thus clinical diagnosis of heart failure is based on the clinical assessment of patient's prior clinical history and reported symptoms combined with the observation of signs derived from a thorough physical examination and selected laboratory and imaging tests. Establishing the subtype of heart failure (HFpEF, HFrEF, HFmrEF), further requires the application of ESC criteria described in Chapter 1.

History

It is crucial to obtain a detailed history to ascertain the presence or absence of possible causes of cardiac damage.[2] Heart failure is much less likely in the absence of a relevant medical history suggesting an increased risk of cardiac damage, compared to the patient with significant risk factors such as previous myocardial infarction.[2–3] In advanced economies nearly 60% of patients diagnosed with acute heart failure have underlying coronary artery disease[4] and, in patients with acute coronary syndromes, myocardial ischemia is often a precipitant factor, especially for *de novo* acute heart failure.[5]

Thus details derived from an accurate clinical history should be taken into account especially known risk factors for the development of heart failure. A prior diagnosis of heart failure, diabetes, hypertension, valvular heart disease, advanced age, male sex, and obesity have all been found to predict the fluid or volume overload typical of congestive heart failure.[6,7] For these reasons, the first diagnostic step is to assess the probability of heart failure and this consists of the evaluation of a potential history of coronary artery disease, arterial hypertension, diuretic use, orthopnoea/paroxysmal nocturnal dyspnea, and other conditions (Table 3.1). Knowledge of the precipitating causes may also have therapeutic and prognostic implications.

Clinical evaluation of symptoms and signs

As described in Chapter 1, heart failure is characterised by dyspnoea, fatigue and signs of volume overload, which may include peripheral edema and pulmonary rales. These symptoms and signs are often the consequence of systemic and pulmonary congestion, due to high left ventricular filling pressures. Even in the absence of overt clinical congestion (with elevation of left ventricular end-diastolic pressure), haemodynamic congestion may also occur, sometimes preceding overt clinical congestion.[4] Notably, while the severity of many other symptoms need not necessarily implicate a poor prognosis,[4] patients with clinical or haemodynamic congestion have worse mortality and rehospitalisation rates.[8–10]

Several tools may be used for the assessment of pulmonary congestion. In clinical practice, the use of cardiac catheterization – the gold standard for the assessment of left-side congestion – is hindered by its invasive nature, and less invasive measures are therefore preferred. Among these, physical examination, body weight, serum sodium, natriuretic peptides and chest X-ray are useful tools for the diagnosis.[4] Newer techniques such as lung ultrasound and impedance monitoring show potential, but have not yet established their position in routine clinical practice.

Beyond the identification of signs of congestion, the evaluation of volume status and peripheral perfusion is pivotal for the diagnosis of heart failure, especially in the acute setting.[1] Given that heart failure is classically characterised by low cardiac output and high filling pressures, an objective measure of volume status is a useful indicators as to the likelihood of the diagnosis.[7] An accurate estimation of volume status is especially critical in the early management of acute heart failure patients.[7] However, assessing volume overload is challenging for the clinician. Errors at this stage often lead to an inappropriate therapy plan and may even increase the risk of mortality.[11] Beyond the baseline evaluation, volume status and peripheral perfusion must be monitored over time. Follow-up assessments of all these parameters will give important warnings on the patient response to treatment, possibly providing the background for modifying treatment.[1]

Some symptoms of heart failure such as peripheral oedema, dyspnoea on exertion and fatigue may not be so helpful for the clinician in making a differential diagnosis, as they are relatively non-specific.[12,3,5] Orthopnoea and paroxysmal nocturnal dyspnoea are more typical of heart failure, but are less common and, therefore, less sensitive.[7] Signs such as an audible third heart sound (S3), displacement of the apical impulse and elevated jugular venous pressure are specific for heart failure, but their identification is more difficult[4] and reproducibility is poor.[5,13] Also signs of fluid retention may disappear soon after diuretic therapy.[1]

Finally, in some groups such as the obese, the elderly and chronic lung disease patients, the identification of symptoms and signs is even more difficult.[14–16] Notably, comorbidities may further complicate the diagnosis. In these cases, rapid objective measures of volume status are needed.[7]

Physical examination

In a case of suspected heart failure, physical examination should consist of the following elements: observation of the patient, palpation and auscultation of the heart, examination of vital signs, heart and lungs as well as neck veins.[8,9,5,4] Additional physical examination may include evaluation of the abdomen and extremities.[2] In particular, jugular venous distention, the presence of rales, and lower extremity oedema are evaluated.[7] The presence of pulmonary rales, jugular venous distention, hepatojugular reflux and pitting peripheral oedema is suggestive of volume overload and therefore increases the likelihood of a diagnosis of heart failure.[17,4] On the other hand it should be noted that the diagnosis of heart failure is not necessarily ruled out if these indicators are not present.[4]

Laboratory assessment

Laboratory testing is recommended by the ESC guidelines as part of the routine diagnostic process in the case of suspected heart failure. Such laboratory investigations can also direct the clinician to explore alternative diagnoses and highlight potentially modifiable causes of heart failure.[4,5] As aforementioned, plasma NPs should be measured after the first diagnostic steps shown in Table 3.1 and Figure 3.1. According to the ESC guidelines, the measurement of NPs should be used to rule out heart failure, and not to establish the diagnosis. Other laboratory exams that should be performed primarily to rule out heart failure are listed in Table 3.1.

Cardiac imaging

The role of cardiac imaging for the diagnosis of heart failure has been well-established. In fact, documentation of an underlying cardiac cause is fundamental to diagnose heart failure. The gold standard for heart failure diagnosis, among the cardiac imaging tools, is echocardiography. This is due to its accuracy, safety, cost-effectiveness and availability.[1]

Echocardiography

Beyond myocardial abnormality, other impairments leading to heart failure may be documented by echocardiography (Table 3.1). For instance, it allows the assessments of chamber volumes, ventricular systolic and diastolic function, wall thickness, valve function, and pulmonary hypertension. Knowledge of these characteristics and of the underlying cardiac problem will also put the background for the treatment plan. In non-acute patients, echocardiography is recommended after the patient is identified as eligible by NP measurement (if the NP level is above the exclusion threshold) or if NP measurement is not available.[1] An early echocardiographic examination is recommended for patients with *de novo* acute heart failure or unknown cardiac function. In high-risk patient groups echocardiography must be performed immediately: patients with haemodynamic instability (particularly in cardiogenic shock) and those suspected of acute life-threatening structural or functional cardiac abnormalities.[1] Echo can be crucial in acute HF, for immediate recognition of treatment options based on clinical phenotypes of AHF.

Other diagnostic tools

A 12-lead electrocardiogram is recommended "in order to determine heart rhythm, heart rate, QRS morphology and QRS duration, and to detect other relevant abnormalities".[1] Electrocardiography will provide additional information for both the diagnosis and the aetiology (e.g. myocardial infarction) and treatment of heart failure. Indeed, heart failure is rarely associated with a totally normal electrocardiogram.[1] Unfortunately, it has been demonstrated that the electrocardiogram has low specificity.[17–18,5] Therefore, it may be used more to exclude a diagnosis of heart failure rather than to establish one.

Chest X-ray, exercise testing, invasive haemodynamic assessments and endomyocardial biopsy are additional tests that may be used in the diagnostic process.[1,2] Lung ultrasound is emerging as a useful test in selected patients for the accurate assessment of pulmonary congestion.[20]

Finally, the role of biomarkers for clinical diagnosis of heart failure is under debate. On the one hand, no clear evidence has been collected to recommend their use in heart failure diagnosis.[1] On the other hand, there are preliminary, encouraging data suggesting their promising use as additional tools in monitoring the progress of clinical cases of heart failure and in the identification of the likely aetiology.

References

1. Ponikowski P, Voors AA, Anker SD, Bueno H, Cleland JG, Coats AJ, Falk V, González-Juanatey JR, Harjola VP, Jankowska EA, Jessup M, Linde C, Nihoyannopoulos P, Parissis JT, Pieske B, Riley JP, Rosano GM, Ruilope LM, Ruschitzka F, Rutten FH, van der Meer P; Authors/Task Force Members; Document Reviewers. 2016 ESC Guidelines for the diagnosis and treatment of acute and chronic heart failure. Eur J Heart Fail. 2016 May 20. doi:10.1002/ejhf.592.
2. Nardone, D. A. (2006). Review: Medical history, physical examination, and routine tests are useful for diagnosing heart failure in dyspnoea. Evid Based Med. 11(3): 72; author reply 72.
3. Mant, J., J. Doust, A. Roalfe, P. Barton, M. R. Cowie, P. Glasziou, D. Mant, R. J. McManus, R. Holder, J. Deeks, K. Fletcher, M. Qume, S. Sohanpal, S. Sanders and F. D. Hobbs (2009). Systematic review and individual patient data meta-analysis of diagnosis of heart failure, with modelling of implications of different diagnostic strategies in primary care. Health Technol Assess. 13(32): 1–207, iii.
4. Kakouros, N. S. and S. N. Kakouros (2015). Clinical Assessment in Acute Heart Failure. Hellenic J Cardiol. 56(4): 285–301.
5. Kelder, J. C., M. J. Cramer, J. van Wijngaarden, R. van Tooren, A. Mosterd, K. G. Moons, J. W. Lammers, M. R. Cowie, D. E. Grobbee and A. W. Hoes (2011). The diagnostic value of physical examination and additional testing in primary care patients with suspected heart failure. Circulation. 124(25): 2865–2873.
6. Wong, G. C. and N. T. Ayas (2007). Clinical approaches to the diagnosis of acute heart failure. Curr Opin Cardiol. 22(3): 207–213.
7. Peacock, W. F. and K. M. Soto (2010). Current techniques of fluid status assessment. Contrib Nephrol. 164: 128–142.
8. Leier, C. V. and K. Chatterjee (2007). The physical examination in heart failure – Part I. Congest Heart Fail. 13(1): 41–47.

9. Leier, C. V. and K. Chatterjee (2007). The physical examination in heart failure – Part II. Congest Heart Fail. 13(2): 99–104.
10. Damy, T., A. Kallvikbacka-Bennett, J. Zhang, K. Goode, L. Buga, J. Hobkirk, A. Yassin, J. L. Dubois-Rande, L. Hittinger, J. G. Cleland and A. L. Clark (2011). Does the physical examination still have a role in patients with suspected heart failure? Eur J Heart Fail. 13(12): 1340–1348.
11. Wuerz, R. C. and S. A. Meador (1992). Effects of prehospital medications on mortality and length of stay in congestive heart failure. Ann Emerg Med. 21(6): 669–674.
12. Davie, A. P., C. M. Francis, L. Caruana, G. R. Sutherland and J. J. McMurray (1997). Assessing diagnosis in heart failure: which features are any use? QJM. 90(5): 335–339.
13. van Riet, E. E., A. W. Hoes, A. Limburg, M. A. Landman, H. van der Hoeven and F. H. Rutten (2014). Prevalence of unrecognized heart failure in older persons with shortness of breath on exertion. Eur J Heart Fail. 16(7): 772–777.
14. Rutten, F. H., K. G. Moons, M. J. Cramer, D. E. Grobbee, N. P. Zuithoff, J. W. Lammers and A. W. Hoes (2005). Recognising heart failure in elderly patients with stable chronic obstructive pulmonary disease in primary care: cross sectional diagnostic study. BMJ. 331(7529): 1379.
15. Daniels, L. B., P. Clopton, V. Bhalla, P. Krishnaswamy, R. M. Nowak, J. McCord, J. E. Hollander, P. Duc, T. Omland, A. B. Storrow, W. T. Abraham, A. H. Wu, P. G. Steg, A. Westheim, C. W. Knudsen, A. Perez, R. Kazanegra, H. C. Herrmann, P. A. McCullough and A. S. Maisel (2006). How obesity affects the cut-points for B-type natriuretic peptide in the diagnosis of acute heart failure. Results from the Breathing Not Properly Multinational Study. Am Heart J. 151(5): 999–1005.
16. Hawkins, N. M., M. C. Petrie, P. S. Jhund, G. W. Chalmers, F. G. Dunn and J. J. McMurray (2009). Heart failure and chronic obstructive pulmonary disease: diagnostic pitfalls and epidemiology. Eur J Heart Fail. 11(2): 130–139.
17. Caldentey, G., P. Khairy, D. Roy, H. Leduc, M. Talajic, N. Racine, M. White, E. O'Meara, M. C. Guertin, J. L. Rouleau and A. Ducharme (2014). Prognostic value of the physical examination in patients with heart failure and atrial fibrillation: insights from the AF-CHF trial (atrial fibrillation and chronic heart failure). JACC Heart Fail. 2(1): 15–23.
18. Davie, A. P., C. M. Francis, M. P. Love, L. Caruana, I. R. Starkey, T. R. Shaw, G. R. Sutherland and J. J. McMurray (1996). Value of the electrocardiogram in identifying heart failure due to left ventricular systolic dysfunction. BMJ. 312(7025): 222.
19. Thomas, J. T., R. F. Kelly, S. J. Thomas, T. D. Stamos, K. Albasha, J. E. Parrillo and J. E. Calvin (2002). Utility of history, physical examination, electrocardiogram, and chest radiograph for differentiating normal from decreased systolic function in patients with heart failure. Am J Med. 112(6): 437–445.
20. Volpicelli G, Elbarbary M, Blaivas M, Lichtenstein DA, Mathis G, Kirkpatrick AW, Melniker L, Gargani L, Noble VE, Via G, Dean A, Tsung JW, Soldati G, Copetti R, Bouhemad B, Reissig A, Agricola E, Rouby J-J, Arbelot C, Liteplo A, Sargsyan A, Silva F, Hoppmann R, Breitkreutz R, Seibel A, Neri L, Storti E, Petrovic T. International evidence-based recommendations for point-of-care lung ultrasound. Intensive Care Med. 2012; 38: 577–591.

4

Medical treatment of heart failure with reduced ejection fraction – prognostic indication

Research on medical interventions that may improve prognosis in patients with chronic heart failure has had great successes in the past decades. Therefore, there are well-established classes of drugs – ACEi, beta-blockers, MRAs – that should be used as first line treatment in all patients with heart failure.[1] In the past few years newer therapeutic approaches have been shown to improve prognosis in patients with heart failure but, since the evidence generated by these newer classes of drugs is less than that of the first three classes of drugs these therapies should be implemented only after an initial treatment with the first line drugs has been implemented.

The main goals of medical therapy in heart failure are to prevent hospital admissions and to improve survival.[1] Because of detrimental effects on long term outcomes seen with some previously studied drugs despite showing promising effects on surrogate end points it has been required, by the main regulatory agencies (EMA and FDA), that all drugs before being approved for the treatment of heart failure were required to show a benefit on mortality and morbidity.[1]

Numbers Needed to Treat (NNT) have been used in the past to indicate the effectiveness of a given treatment. However, since treatments approved for the treatment of heart failure have been tested in different time periods and using different background therapies NNT will not be used in this book in order to avoid unfair comparisons between treatments that have not been tested head to head.

Neurohumoral antagonist drugs acting on the Renin Angiotensin Aldosterone

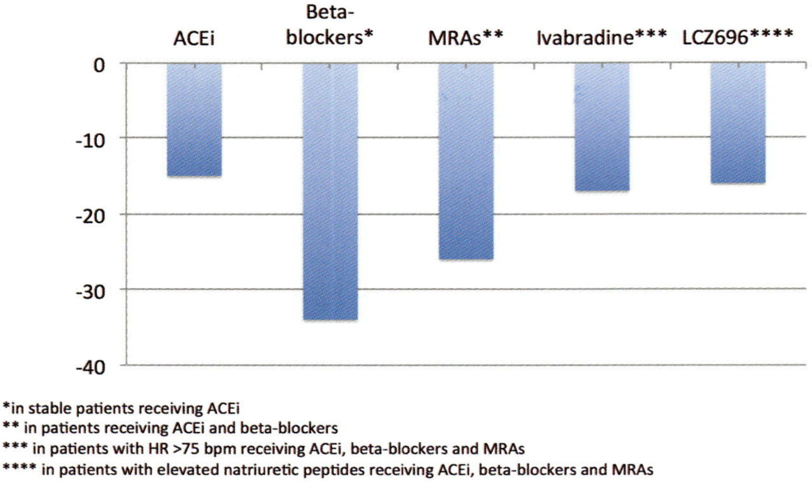

FIGURE 4.1 Drugs that reduce mortality in heart failure with reduced ejection fraction

System [ACE inhibitors MRAs and a dual vasopeptidase inhibitor] and on the Sympathetic Nervous Control of the cardiovascular system [beta-adrenergic blockers] have been shown to improve survival in patients with systolic HF and should be considered at different stages in the treatment of every patient. Drugs acting on the sequaele of neurohormonal activation such as the heart rate reducing agent ivabradine have also been shown to improve mortality and should also be considered when appropriate. These medications should be considered in all patients with chronic heart failure in conjunction with a diuretic when there is the need to relieve the symptoms and signs of congestion.[2–16] (Figure 4.1). Angiotensin II type I receptor blockers are often considered equivalent to ACEi but since they did not show any effect on overall mortality in patients with HFrEF, their use should be limited only to those patients intolerant of an ACE-inhibitor.[17–18]

Angiotensin-converting enzyme inhibitors [ACEi]

There is overwhelming evidence to support the use of ACEi in patients with heart failure. ACEi have been shown to reduce mortality and morbidity in patients with all different forms of heart failure and reduced ejection fraction (post-infarction, post-acute, chronic, left ventricular dysfunction).[2–4] Therefore, ACEi must always be considered in all patients with heart failure, NYHA class I-IV and an LVEF < 40%.[1]

Given their mortality benefit ACEi must represent the initial therapeutic choice, alone or in association with a diuretic, and their dose should be up-titrated to the evidence-based dose or, in any case to the maximum tolerated dose in order to achieve an adequate inhibition of RAAS.[3]

ACEi may increase K+ levels and therefore caution should be posed when they are administered to patients with elevated K+ levels while they are contra-indicated in patients with moderate hyperkalaemia (K+ > 6.0 mmol/L). Drugs or substances that increase K+ plasma levels such as K+ supplements and K+-sparing diuretics, e.g. amiloride and triamterene, may potentiate the effect of ACEi on K+ and their use must be restricted when an increase in K+ is observed. Dose adjustment may be needed in patients with severe renal dysfunction (eGFR < 30 mL/min/1.73 m^2) and in those with arterial hypotension (systolic blood pressure < 90 mmHg).

Beta-Blockers

The pivotal trials with beta-blockers in heart failure were conducted in symptomatic patients despite treatment with an ACE inhibitor and, in most cases, a diuretic.[5–11] Although these treatments are regarded as complementary and most often a beta-blocker and an ACE inhibitor are started together after diagnosis of HFrEF there is no trial evidence to support this practice. Studies aiming at implementing beta-blockers before adequate up-titration of an ACEi have shown an increase in hospitalisations for heart failure.[10] Unlike ACEi, Beta-blockers should be initiated in clinically stable NYHA Class II-IV patients with LVEF <40%. Implementation of beta-blockers in patients not receiving adequate ACEi has been shown to increase hospitalisation rates. Therefore, it is not recommended to start a beta-blocker before having started an ACEi. However, there is agreement in the guidelines that beta-blockers and ACEIs can be started together in stable patients.[1]

The striking effect of beta-blockers in reducing the risk of sudden cardiac death and overall mortality observed in the past should be nowadays be reconsidered given the use of ICDs. It is most probable that the overall effect of beta-blockers on mortality will be maintained but the size of the effect will be probably lower than that predicted by the early studies in patients not having an ICD implanted.

It must be noted that most beta-blocker trials included patients with heart failure who were younger (mean age 61–64) than those seen in clinical practice (mean age >70). Furthermore, large international surveys have shown that only a minority of patients with heart failure receive beta-blockers at a dose that is recommended as target. This under-dosing may reflect a lack of tolerability in

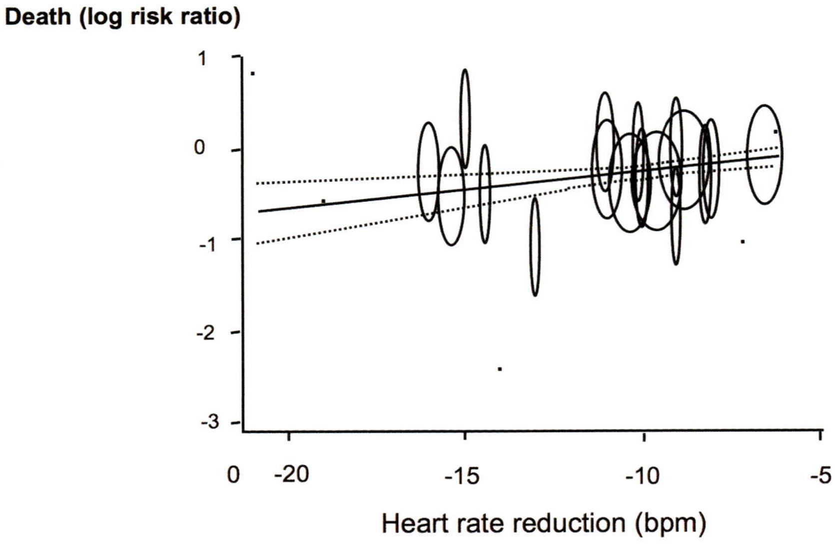

FIGURE 4.2 Relation between the magnitude of heart rate reduction and outcomes in heart failure (McAliser FA et al. *Ann Intern Med*. 2009: 150: 784–94)

patients who are typically relatively old and have co-morbidities. However, the CIBIS-ELD study showed that only 20% of patients randomised to carvedilol or bisoprolol may tolerate full dose beta-blockade.[19]

Several meta-analyses have shown that the prognostic effect of beta-blockers is not related to the dose but to the degree of heart rate reduction supporting the prognostic importance of heart rate in heart failure (see Figure 4.2).

Recently, an individual patient meta-analysis of the large randomised placebo controlled studies has shown that beta-blockers have a neutral effect on mortality and morbidity in patients with HFrEF and atrial fibrillation.[20] Therefore, beta-blockers should only be considered for rate control in patients with HFrEF who are in AF. Their benefit is likely to be greater in those with high (>110 bpm) heart rate. Because of their anti-ischaemic effect beta-blockers should be always considered in patients with an ischaemic origin of HF.

Beta-blockers are contra-indicated in patients with symptomatic bradycardia and in those with second- or third-degree AV block unless they have been implanted with a permanent pacemaker. Beta-blockers are also contraindicated in patients with significant peripheral arterial disease and in those with critical limb ischaemia and in those with asthma or with a history of asthma. Although the new ESC/HFA guidelines suggest that if cardio-selective beta-blockers are indicated, asthma is not necessarily an absolute contraindication, the benefit/risk of these drugs in this class of patients is negative. Chronic

Obstructive Pulmonary Disease is not a contra-indication for the use of beta-blockers in patients with heart failure.

Beta-blockers should be used with caution in patients with recent (< 4 weeks) exacerbation of heart failure (e.g. current or recent hospital admission with worsening HF), and in those with severe heart failure (NYHA class IV). In patients with signs of congestion – i.e. hypotension systolic < 90 mmHg, ascites, raised JVP, peripheral oedema – congestion should be relieved and 'euvolaemia' should be achieved before starting a beta-blocker.

In beta-blocker naïve patients it is always advisable to start with a low dose and to double the dose slowly at not less than 2-week intervals monitoring heart rate, blood pressure, and clinical status. When starting beta-blockers or during the up-titration phase it is important to detect potential clinical deterioration. Therefore, patients should be encouraged to weigh themselves daily in the morning after waking and to report any persistent weight increase of > 1.5–2.0 kg/day. In elderly and fragile patients as in patients with more advanced stages of heart failure a slower up-titration may be needed. Beta-blockers may induce fatigue through several mechanisms. If fatigue occurs the dose of beta-blocker should be halved.

Mineralocorticoid/aldosterone receptor antagonists [MRAs]

MRAs are drugs that block the receptors that bind aldosterone. First and second generation MRAs also bind, with different degree of affinity corticosteroid and sex steroid receptors. Newer MRAs have high affinity to block aldosterone receptors. Spironolactone and Eplerenone have been shown to reduce mortality and events in patients with HFrEF treated with an ACEi and a beta-blocker.[12–13] Potassium canrenoate is an active metabolite of spironolactone approved in some European Countries for the treatment of patients with HFrEF and it is the metabolite responsible for most of the pharmacodynamic effect of spironolactone.

MRAs are recommended in all symptomatic (NYHA II-IV) patients with HFrEF (LVEF ≤ 35%) already receiving an ACEi and a beta-blocker in order to reduce mortality and HF hospitalization.[1,12–13]

MRAs are well tolerated and the occurrence of hyperkalaemia has been low in the randomised studies conducted with spironolactone and eplerenone. It is advisable, however, to start MRAs after having checked renal function and electrolytes (particularly K+), starting with a low dose (see above) and should be up-titrated after 4–8 weeks after having checked K+ levels. Thereafter, K+ levels should be checked at 12 weeks; 6, 9, and 12 months and 4-monthly thereafter. A closer monitoring may be needed in patients with borderline high K+ levels. MRAs should be used with caution in patients with impaired renal function (eGFR < 60 mL/min/1.73 m^2) and in those with elevated serum potassium levels (> 5.0 mmol/L). The dose of MRAs should be halved if K+ rises above 5.5 mmol/L or eGFR <30 mL/min/1.73 m^2. MRAs should be stopped and adequate measures should be undertaken if K+ rises to >6.0 mmol/L or eGFR <20 mL/min/1.73 m^2.

Ivabradine

Ivabradine is a drug that slows heart rate through inhibition of the If channel in the sinus node. The net effect of ivabradine is a prolongation of diastole with a prolongation of diastolic filling period. Unlike beta-blockers this effect is obtained with a preservation of ventricular relaxation and with lower left ventricular end diastolic pressures. Because of its specific effect on the sinus node ivabradine should only be used in patients in sinus rhythm.

Ivabradine reduced the combined endpoint of mortality and hospitalization for HF in patients symptomatic HFrEF with LVEF ≤ 35% in the SHIFT study (see Figure 4.3).[14–15] The benefits have been shown in patients often receiving treatment with a beta-blocker, an ACEI (or ARB), and an MRA. The SHIFT study has shown that the mortality benefit of ivabradine is related to its heart rate reducing effect and that is greatest in patients achieving a heart rate <60 bpm.[21] The combined analysis of the SHIFT study in patients with

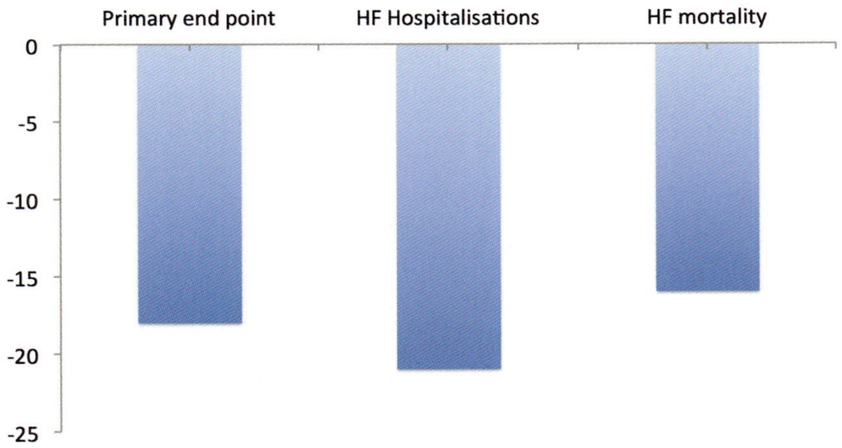

FIGURE 4.3 Effect of ivabradine on mortality and morbidity in patients with HFrEF (Svedberg K et al. *Lancet.* 2010 Sep 11: 376(9744): 875–885)

HFrEF and of the Beautiful study in patients with ischaemic left ventricular dysfunction have shown that treatment with ivabradine was associated with significant relative risk reductions in cardiovascular outcomes including 13% relative risk reduction for the composite of cardiovascular mortality and 19% for HF hospitalization alone. The analysis also showed significant relative risk reductions for the composite of cardiovascular mortality, HF hospitalizations, or myocardial infarction (MI); cardiovascular mortality and non-fatal MI; and MI hospitalization.[22] These findings support the importance of treatment with ivabradine for improvement of clinical outcomes in patients with LV dysfunction whether or not presenting with heart failure.

The international guidelines have acknowledged the prognostic benefits of ivabradine and indicate the drug for the treatment of patients treated with an ACEi, a beta-blocker and a MRA with left ventricular dysfunction and those with Class (II-IV) HFrEF (LVEF <35%) with heart rate > 70 bpm to reduce heart failure hospitalisations and cardiovascular mortality.[1]

In patients with HFrEF with a LVEF ≤ 35% who are unable to tolerate or have contra-indications for a beta-blocker, ivabradine should be considered to reduce the risk of heart failure hospitalizations and cardiovascular death.

The European Medicines Agency has requested an analysis of the SHIFT trial with ivabradine in order to identify the heart rate threshold above which ivabradine confers a survival benefit and it was found that the mortality benefit of ivabradine is apparent for heart rates ≥ 75 bpm, with a 17% reduction in overall mortality and a 39% reduction in death from heart failure (see

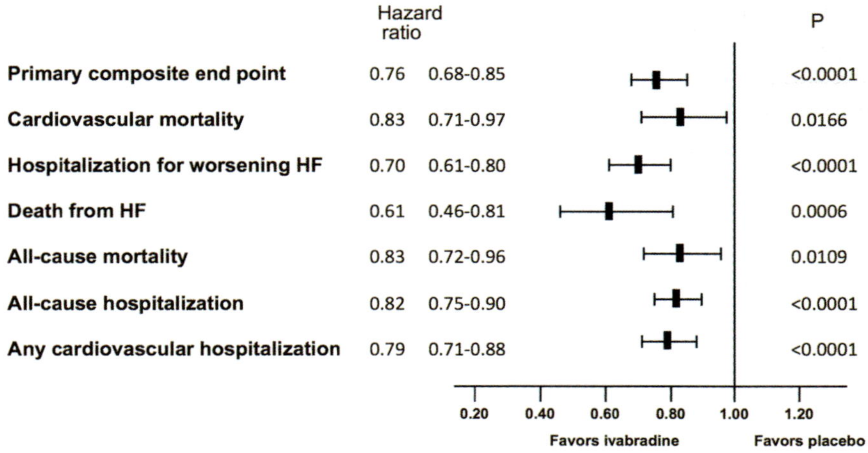

FIGURE 4.4 Effect of ivabradine on outcomes in patients with HFrEF and HR ≥75 bpm (Böhm M et al. *Clin Res Cardiol.* 2012)

Figure 4.4). Ivabradine is very safe to use and has few drug to drug interactions, however, caution should be exercised in patients developing resting heart rate < 50 bpm during treatment and in those with liver dysfunction. Ivabradine should not be used in patients receiving verapamil, or diltiazem. However, these two drugs are contraindicated in HFrEF anyway.

Studies in patients receiving beta-blockers have shown that the association of ivabradine and a beta-blocker is more effective than increasing the dose of the beta-blocker in achieving target heart rate, improving exercise capacity and functional performance. Therefore, ivabradine/beta-blockade is to be preferred to a full implementation of beta-blocker alone.

Treatment with ivabradine should be started at 5 mg twice daily and the dose should be stepped up after 2–4 weeks, if target heart rate has not been reached, to the target dose of 7.5 mg twice daily.

ARNI - angiotensin receptor neprilysin inhibitor

ARNI is a new therapeutic class of drugs that block the angiotensin II type 1 receptor and inhibit the neutral endopeptidase system. This latter system degrades natriuretic peptides and bradykinin together with other peptides. The first in class is LCZ696 that is a molecule that combines the moieties of Valsartan and Sucubutril in one single drug substance. LCZ696 simultaneously blocks the angiotensin II type 1 receptors and increases circulating levels of A-type natriuretic peptide (ANP) and B type natriuretic peptide (BNP). The increased NP levels enhance diuresis, natriuresis, and myocardial relaxation and inhibit renin and aldosterone secretion. LCZ696 is the first molecule of this class and has been developed by co-crystallization of valsartan and sacubitril in one single agent.

The PARADIGM-HF study compared the long-term effects of LCZ696 with those of Enalapril on mortality and morbidity in patients with ambulatory, symptomatic HFrEF with LVEF ≤ 35% (only a small minority of patients with LVEF <40% were included in the early phases of the study), elevated plasma NP levels (BNP ≥ 150 pg/mL or NT-proBNP ≥ 600 pg/mL or a BNP ≥ 100 pg/mL or NT-proBNP ≥ 400 pg/mL if they had been hospitalized for HF within the previous 12 months), an estimated GFR (eGFR) ≥ 30 mL/min/1.73 m^2 of body surface area, who were able to tolerate enalapril 10 mg b.i.d.[16]

In these patients LCZ696 reduced the composite end point of death from cardiovascular causes or hospitalization for heart failure by 20%, death by 16% and need for hospitalisation by 21% (see Figure 4.5). For these reasons LCZ696 is recommended by the ESC/HFA guidelines for the treatment of out of hospital patients with HFrEF who remain symptomatic despite the

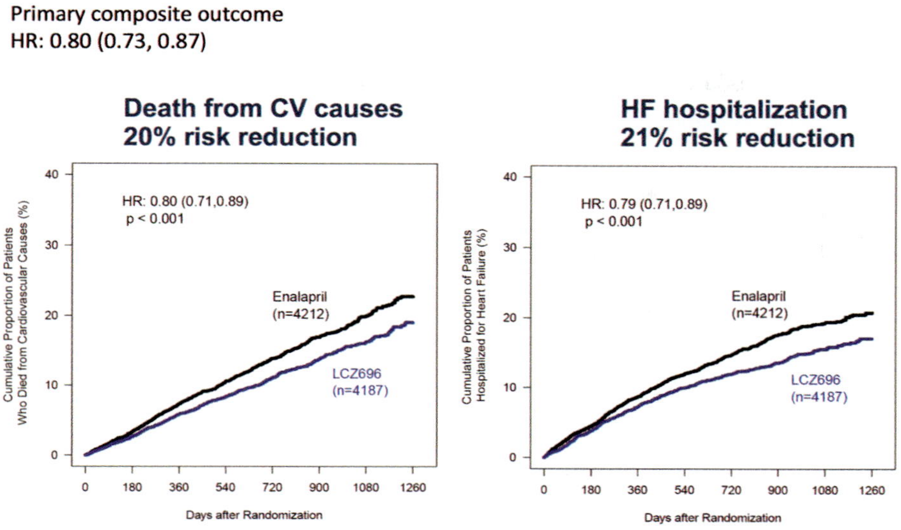

FIGURE 4.5 Effect of LCZ696 on the components of the primary end point in the PARADIGM-HF study

treatment with an ACEi a beta-blocker and an MRA that also have elevated natriuretic peptides and are able to tolerate 10 mg bid of enalapril.

The recommended starting dose of LCZ696 is 100 mg (49 mg/51 mg) twice daily, the dose should be doubled at 2–4 weeks to the target dose of 200 mg (97 mg/103 mg) twice daily if tolerated. If patients experience low systolic blood pressure ≤95 mmHg, symptomatic hypotension, hyperkalaemia, or renal dysfunction, adjustment of concomitant medicinal products, or down–titration or discontinuation of LCZ696 is recommended. Treatment with LCZ696 should not be initiated in patients with serum potassium level >5.4 mmol/l or with SBP <100 mmHg.

LCZ696 may induce symptomatic hypotension, especially in the elderly and for this reason caution in its uptitration should be exercised in patients with low blood pressure levels. The PARADIGM-HF study reduced the likelihood of angioedema with LCZ696 by recruiting only those patients who tolerated ACEi therapy and, given the absence of safety data in ACEi naïve patients the drug should not be used in ACEi naïve patients and ACEIs should be withheld for at least 36 hours before initiating LCZ696.

ARBs – Angiotensin II type I receptor blockers and double RAAS blockade

The role of ARBs in the treatment of patients with HFrEF has changed in the past few years and now, in line with the scientific evidence ARBs are only recommended as an alternative in those few patients who are intolerant to an ACE inhibitor.[1] The CHARM programme showed that Candesartan was able to reduce cardiovascular mortality, but not overall mortality, in patients with HF.[17] On the other hand the Val-HEFT study showed that Valsartan had only a marginal effect on heart failure hospitalisations (but not on the overall days in hospital) in patients with HFrEF.[18] A meta-analysis including 33 randomised controlled trials with 68 405 patients (mean age 61 years, 71% men) and mean duration of 52 weeks showed that while dual blockade (ACEi+ARB) of the RAAS was not associated with a clinical benefit in reducing all cause mortality (relative risk [RR] = 0.97; 95% CI 0.89–1.06) and cardiovascular mortality (RR = 0.96; 0.88–1.05) compared with monotherapy, it was only associated with a reduction in heart failure hospitalisations (RR = 0.82, 0.74–0.92) and with an increased risk of hyperkalaemia (RR = 1.55; 1.32–1.82), hypotension (RR = 1.66; 1.38–1.98) and renal failure (RR = 1.41; 1.09–1.84) thereby suggesting that dual blockade of the renin-angiotensin system is associated with an excessive risk of adverse events not balanced by an effect on mortality or on hospitalisations.[23] The EMA suggested that the benefits of double RAAS blockade outweigh risk only in a selected group of patients with HFrEF in whom other treatments are unsuitable. The ESC/HFA guidelines on heart failure suggest that ARBs are only indicated for the treatment of patients with HFrEF who cannot tolerate an ACEI because of serious side effects and that the combination of ACEI/ARBs should be limited only to symptomatic patients with HFrEF who are unable to tolerate an MRA. In this case the double blockade of the RAAS must be used under strict supervision.

Metabolic agents

Trimetazidine is a metabolic modulator that blocks free fatty acid oxidation and improves glucose oxidation thereby improving the metabolic efficiency of the heart. Trimetazidine has been tested in several small studies in patients with HFrEF. Three meta-analyses of the available data suggest that Trimetazidine may improve prognosis in patients with HFrEF.[24–26] Trimetazidine is therefore indicated where appropriate in patients with HFrEF. A specific benefit of trimetazidine is observed in patients with an ischaemic origin of left ventricular dysfunction as well as in the elderly and in diabetic patients.[27–30]

Diuretics

Diuretics reduce signs and symptoms of congestion in patients with HFrEF. Although their effects on mortality and morbidity have not been formally tested in a randomised controlled study, a meta-analysis has shown that in patients with chronic HFrEF loop and thiazide diuretics reduce the risk of death and worsening HF compared to placebo.[31]

Different diuretics have different effects with loop diuretics having a shorter but stronger diuresis than thiazides and the combination may be used to treat resistant oedema. Since the main aim of diuretic therapy is to reduce congestion and maintain euvolaemia the dose should be adjusted over time. Although in selected cases patients and can be trained to self-adjust their diuretic dose, the adjustment should be in the majority of cases supervised by a healthcare professional. More recently new subcutaneous delivery systems of diuretics have been developed for easier titration of diuretic dose in patients with the more advanced stages of the disease.

Therefore, the treatment of patients with HFrEF should be implemented gradually through steps that take into account the prognostic benefits of the different classes of drugs. Diuretics should always be used for the control of fluid balance and their dose should be appropriately adjusted according to patient conditions in order to maintain euvolaemia. The initial step of the treatment of patients with HFrEF should include ACEi and beta-blockers taking into account that beta-blockers can be started together with ACEi but not before ACEi had been started. Beta-blockers should be used only in NYHA class II-III patients and they should not be used in haemodynamically unstable patients, should be used with caution in patients with recent (< 4 weeks) exacerbation of heart failure or in those with signs of congestion or hypotension. In the few patients that have intolerance to ACEi an ARB may be considered.

These drugs should be titrated to the maximum tolerated dose. If symptoms persist an MRA must be considered carefully monitoring electrolytes. If the patient is still symptomatic ivabradine and LCZ696 should be considered. These two drugs are not alternative but may be complementary as ivabradine can be safely started in all patients in sinus rhythm where it is indicated and in all those many patients with low blood pressure values that may need to down-titrate beta-blockers dose in order to be able to receive LCZ696.

References

1. Ponikowski P, Voors A, Anker S et al The Task Force for the diagnosis and treatment of acute and chronic heart failure of the European Society of Cardiology (ESC). 2016 ESC Guidelines for the diagnosis and treatment of acute and chronic heart failure. European Journal of Heart Failure. Published online 26 May 2016.
2. Garg R, Yusuf S. Overview of randomized trials of angiotensin-converting enzyme inhibitors on mortality and morbidity in patients with heart failure. JAMA. 1995; 273: 1450–1456.
3. Packer M, Poole-Wilson PA, Armstrong PW, Cleland JGF, Horowitz JD, Massie BM, Ryden L, Thygesen K, Uretsky BF, Ryde´n L, Thygesen K, Uretsky BF, ATLAS Study Group. Comparative effects of low and high doses of the angiotensin-converting enzyme inhibitor, lisinopril, on morbidity and mortality in chronic heart failure. Circulation. 1999; 100: 2312–2318.
4. SOLVD Investigattors. Effect of enalapril on survival in patients with reduced left ventricular ejection fractions and congestive heart failure. N Engl J Med. 1991; 325: 293–302.
5. Hjalmarson A, Goldstein S, Fagerberg B, Wedel H, Waagstein F, Kjekshus J, Wikstrand J, ElAllaf D, V´ıtovec J, Aldershvile J, Halinen M, Dietz R, Neuhaus KL, Ja´nosi A, Thorgeirsson G, Dunselman PH, Gullestad L, Kuch J, Herlitz J, Rickenbacher P, Ball S, Gottlieb S, Deedwania P. MERIT-HF Study Group. Effects of controlled-release metoprolol on total mortality, hospitalizations, and well-being in patients with heart failure: the Metoprolol CR/XL Randomized Intervention Trial in congestive Heart Failure (MERIT-HF). JAMA. 2000; 283: 1295–1302.
6. Packer M, Coats AJ, Fowler MB, Katus HA, Krum H, Mohacsi P, Rouleau JL, Tendera M, Castaigne A, Roecker EB, Schultz MK, DeMets DL. Effect of carvedilol on survival in severe chronic heart failure. N Engl J Med. 2001; 344: 1651–1658.
7. Effect of metoprolol CR/XL in chronic heart failure: Metoprolol CR/XL Randomised Intervention Trial in Congestive Heart Failure (MERIT-HF). Lancet. 1999; 353: 2001–2007.
8. Packer M. Effect of carvedilol on the morbidity of patients with severe chronic heart failure: results of the Carvedilol Prospective Randomized Cumulative Survival (COPERNICUS) Study. Circulation. 2002; 106: 2194–2199.
9. CIBIS-II Investigators and Committees. The Cardiac Insufficiency Bisoprolol Study II (CIBIS-II): a randomised trial. Lancet. 1999; 353: 9–13.
10. Willenheimer R, van Veldhuisen DJ, Silke B, Erdmann E, Follath F, Krum H, Ponikowski P, Skene A, van de Ven L, Verkenne P, Lechat P, CIBIS III Investigators. Effect on survival and hospitalization of initiating treatment for chronic heart failure with bisoprolol followed by enalapril, as compared with the opposite sequence: results of the randomized Cardiac Insufficiency Bisoprolol Study (CIBIS) III. Circulation. 2005; 112: 2426–2435.
11. Flather MD, Shibata MC, Coats AJS, Van Veldhuisen DJ, Parkhomenko A, Borbola J, Cohen-Solal A, Dumitrascu D, Ferrari R, Lechat P, Soler-Soler J, Tavazzi L, Spinarova L, Toman J, Boehm M, Anker SD, Thompson SG, Poole-Wilson PA, SENIORS Investigators. Randomized trial to determine the effect of nebivolol on mortality and

cardiovascular hospital admission in elderly patients with heart failure (SENIORS). Eur Heart J. 2005; 26: 215–225.

12. Pitt B, Zannad F, Remme WJ, Cody R, Castaigne A, Perez A, Palensky J, Wittes J. The effect of spironolactone on morbidity and mortality in patients with severe heart failure. N Engl J Med. 1999; 341: 709–717.
13. Zannad F, McMurray JJV, Krum H, Van Veldhuisen DJ, Swedberg K, Shi H, Vincent J, Pocock SJ, Pitt B. Eplerenone in patients with systolic heart failure and mild symptoms. N Engl J Med. 2011; 364: 11–21.
14. Swedberg K, Komajda M, Boehm M, Borer JS, Ford I, Dubost-Brama A, Lerebours G, Tavazzi L. Ivabradine and outcomes in chronic heart failure (SHIFT): a randomised placebo-controlled study. Lancet. 2010; 376: 875–885.
15. Swedberg K, Komajda M, Boehm M, Borer J, Robertson M, Tavazzi L, Ford I. Effects on outcomes of heart rate reduction by ivabradine in patients with congestive heart failure: is there an influence of beta-blocker dose?: findings from the SHIFT (Systolic Heart failure treatment with the I(f) inhibitor ivabradine Trial) study. J Am Coll Cardiol. 2012; 59: 1938–1945.
16. McMurray JJ, Packer M, Desai AS, Gong J, Lefkowitz MP, Rizkala AR, Rouleau JL, Shi VC, Solomon SD, Swedberg K, Zile MR, PARADIGM-HF Investigators and Committees. Angiotensin-neprilysin inhibition versus enalapril in heart failure. N Engl J Med. 2014; 371: 993–1004.
17. Granger CB, McMurray JJV, Yusuf S, Held P, Michelson EL, Olofsson B, Ostergren J, Pfeffer MA, Swedberg K. Effects of candesartan in patients with chronic heart failure and reduced left-ventricular systolic function intolerant to angiotensin-converting-enzyme inhibitors: the CHARM-Alternative trial. Lancet. 2003; 362: 772–776.
18. Cohn JN, Tognoni G. A randomized trial of the angiotensin-receptor blocker valsartan in chronic heart failure. N Engl J Med. 2001; 345: 1667–1675.
19. Düngen HD, Apostolovic S, Inkrot S, Tahirovic E, Töpper A, Mehrhof F, Prettin C, Putnikovic B, Neskovic AN, Krotin M, Sakac D, Lainscak M, Edelmann F, Wachter R, Rau T, Eschenhagen T, Doehner W, Anker SD, Waagstein F, Herrmann-Lingen C, Gelbrich G, Dietz R; CIBIS-ELD investigators and Project Multicentre Trials in the Competence Network Heart Failure. Titration to target dose of bisoprolol vs. carvedilol in elderly patients with heart failure: the CIBIS-ELD trial. Eur J Heart Fail. 2011 Jun; 13(6): 670–80.
20. Kotecha D, Holmes J, Krum H, Altman DG, Manzano L, Cleland JGF, Lip GYH, Coats AJS, Andersson B, Kirchhof P, von Lueder TG, Wedel H, Rosano G, Shibata MC, Rigby A, Flather MD. Efficacy of b blockers in patients with heart failure plus atrial fibrillation: an individual-patient data meta-analysis. Lancet. 2014; 384: 2235–2243.
21. Boehm M, Borer J, Ford I, Gonzalez-Juanatey JR, Komajda M, Lopez-Sendon J, Reil J-C, Swedberg K, Tavazzi L. Heart rate at baseline influences the effect of ivabradine on cardiovascular outcomes in chronic heart failure: analysis from the SHIFT study. Clin Res Cardiol. 2013; 102: 11–22.
22. Fox K, Komajda M, Ford I, Robertson M, Böhm M, Borer JS, Steg PG, Tavazzi L, Tendera M, Ferrari R, Swedberg K. Effect of ivabradine in patients with left-ventricular systolic dysfunction: a pooled analysis of individual patient data from the BEAUTIFUL and SHIFT trials. Eur Heart J. 2013 Aug; 34(29): 2263–70.

23. Makani H, Bangalore S, Desouza KA, Shah A, Messerli FH. Efficacy and safety of dual blockade of the renin-angiotensin system: meta-analysis of randomised trials. BMJ. 2013 Jan 28; 346:f360.
24. Grajek S, Michalak M. The effect of trimetazidine added to pharmacological treatment on all-cause mortality in patients with systolic heart failure. Cardiology. 2015; 131(1): 22–9.
25. Zhang L, Lu Y, Jiang H, Zhang L, Sun A, Zou Y, Ge J. Additional use of trimetazidine in patients with chronic heart failure: a meta-analysis. J Am Coll Cardiol. 2012 Mar 6; 59(10): 913–22.
26. Gao D, Ning N, Niu X, Hao G, Meng Z. Trimetazidine: a meta-analysis of randomised controlled trials in heart failure. Heart. 2011 Feb; 97(4): 278–86.
27. Lopatin YM, Rosano GM, Fragasso G, Lopaschuk GD, Seferovic PM, Gowdak LH, Vinereanu D, Hamid MA, Jourdain P, Ponikowski P. Rationale and benefits of trimetazidine by acting on cardiac metabolism in heart failure. Int J Cardiol. 2016 Jan 15; 203: 909–15.
28. Fragasso G, Rosano G, Baek SH, Sisakian H, Di Napoli P, Alberti L, Calori G, Kang SM, Sahakyan L, Sanosyan A, Vitale C, Marazzi G, Margonato A, Belardinelli R. Effect of partial fatty acid oxidation inhibition with trimetazidine on mortality and morbidity in heart failure: results from an international multicentre retrospective cohort study. Int J Cardiol. 2013 Mar 10; 163(3): 320–5.
29. Iyengar SS, Rosano GM. Effect of antianginal drugs in stable angina on predicted mortality risk after surviving a myocardial infarction: a preliminary study (METRO). Am J Cardiovasc Drugs. 2009; 9(5): 293–7.
29. Marazzi G, Wajngarten M, Vitale C, Patrizi R, Pelliccia F, Gebara O, Pierri H, Ramires JA, Volterrani M, Fini M, Rosano GM. Effect of free fatty acid inhibition on silent and symptomatic myocardial ischemia in diabetic patients with coronary artery disease. Int J Cardiol. 2007 Aug 9; 120(1): 79–84.
30. Vitale C, Wajngaten M, Sposato B, Gebara O, Rossini P, Fini M, Volterrani M, Rosano GM. Trimetazidine improves left ventricular function and quality of life in elderly patients with coronary artery disease. Eur Heart J. 2004 Oct; 25(20): 1814–21.
31. Faris R, Flather M, Purcell H, Henein M, Poole-Wilson P, Coats A. Current evidence supporting the role of diuretics in heart failure: a meta analysis of randomised controlled trials. Int J Cardiol. 2002; 82: 149–158.

5

Medical treatment of heart failure with reduced ejection fraction – improving clinical status and functional capacity

The improvement of functional capacity is one of the main goals of treatment in patients with HFrEF.[1] In the past, despite significant effects on exercise capacity some drugs (e.g. ibopamine, flosequinan) have shown detrimental effects on long-term outcomes in patients with HFrEF.[2,3] It is perhaps notable that both of these drugs had shown signals of increased safety concerns during the earlier clinical phases of their development.[4,5] The challenge is to encourage a timely identification of effective treatments that can enhance functional performance in HF without the more difficult and more expensive path to prove all drugs also reduce mortality. It is valuable to have approved and effective treatments that can do the first without the need for the second in all cases, provided adequate safety can be assured.

It is now clear that stabilisation or improvement of exercise capacity reflects the ability of effective treatments to slow or prevent progressive worsening of HF and are important patient related outcomes. Amongst the drugs effective in improving prognosis in patients with heart failure some have a neutral or sometime negative effect on exercise capacity while some others have shown a significant improvement in exercise capacity. ACEi, ARBs and MRAs have a neutral effect on exercise capacity in patients with HFrEF while beta-blockers tend to reduce exercise tolerance. There are no data available on the effect of LCZ696 on exercise capacity in patients with HFrEF.

The only pharmacological treatments with a significant effect on cardiovascular prognosis that have consistently shown to improve exercise capacity are ivabradine, trimetazidine, intravenous iron and diuretics. Amongst devices

CRT has been consistently shown to improve prognosis and improve exercise capacity in patients with HFrEF, and cardiac contractility modulation (CCM) have been shown to improve exercise capacity in one study and a comprehensive individual patient data meta-analysis.[6–7]

There are no adequate surrogate measures for mortality in heart failure, however once the drug has been shown to have a positive effect on prognosis it is important to assess its effect on well being. This can be difficult because of both patient and researchers biases in assessing well-being. Indeed, patients' perceptions may be affected by their state of health, by their expectations, by related co-morbidities and by their personal priorities. Similarly, the medical assessment of patient general status is influenced consciously or unconsciously by information on the severity of the disease derived from investigations, and the doctors' perceptions of likely prognosis derived from these. Exercise capacity, when reliably measured, represents a good measure of the effect of a given treatment on functional status of patients with heart failure.

Exercise tests using both bicycle or treadmill have been used to assess the effects of therapy in heart failure.[8] More objective assessment of true maximal exercise capacity utilising respiratory gas exchange to establish a close to maximal effort improves reliability of exercise capacity assessment. This allows the assessment of maximal oxygen consumption as the best available measure of functional capacity. This has been used for the pre-transplant assessment of patients with heart failure and assessing the effects of heart failure interventions. However, exercise testing and assessment of gas exchange may be difficult to administer in all patients as patients may be unable to exercise on a bicycle or to breathe into a gas exchange mask. Heart failure patients, however, can perform a self-paced 6 min walk test (6MWT). This test has long been used as an outcome measure in clinical trials and its results have been shown to be concordant with changes in symptoms, suggesting that it is a good indicator for symptom benefit.[8] A significant increase in 6MWT has been observed with cardiac resynchronization and CCM for example.[6–7]

ACE-inhibitors and ARBs

Despite their prognostic benefits ACE inhibitors have failed to show significant effects on functional capacity and no difference between ACE-I and ARBs has been ever demonstrated.

In general the adequately sized studies aimed at assessing the effect of ACE-I on exercise capacity have reported a neutral effect on functional status. One large multicentre, placebo-controlled trial testing captopril and cilazapril failed to show any effect of ACE-inhibition.[9] (Figure 5.1) One study testing the

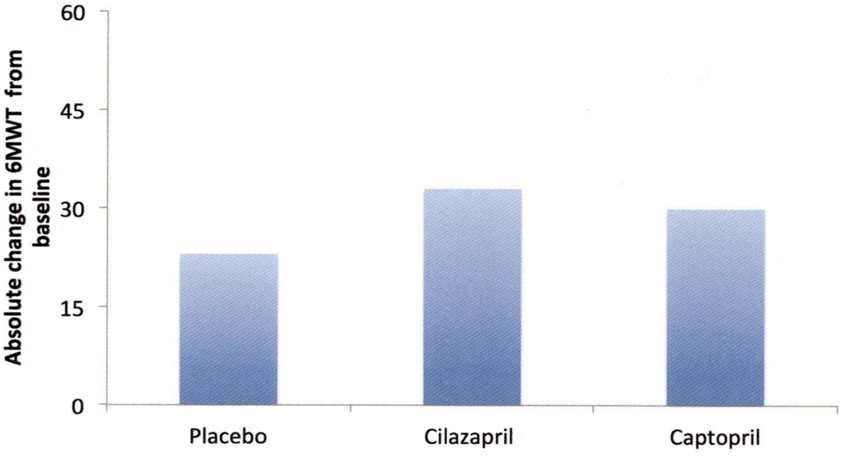

FIGURE 5.1 Effect of ACE inhibitors in HFrEF in the Cilazapril captopril study[9]

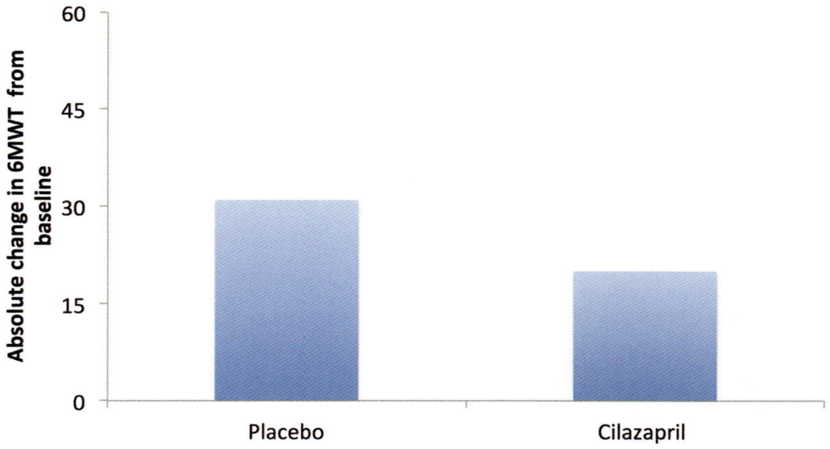

FIGURE 5.2 Effect of candesartan on exercise capacity in HFrEF.[11]

effect of perindopril showed a significant improvement in exercise capacity.[10] One adequately sized study compared candesartan with placebo and showed no effect (Figure 5.2).[11] Four studies have compared the effect of ARBs with the ACEI enalapril, and found no differences in functional capacity nor on patient reported outcomes.[12–15] Therefore, the overall effect of RAAS inhibitors on functional capacity and symptoms appears to be neutral.

Beta-blockers

Beta-blockers have a neutral or negative effect on exercise capacity.[8] A small effect has been shown with carvedilol in some studies but this effect has not been consistently demonstrated and confirmed. Only 3 of 20 trials and only one of five multicentre studies investigating the effect of beta-blockers on 6MWT showed an improvement.[8,16–20] When detected, this effect has been marginal (Figure 5.3). Two trials compared the effect of metoprolol and carvedilol on 6MWT and showed no difference between these two beta-blockers.[21,22] Carvedilol and bisoprolol have consistently been shown to be inferior to ivabradine in their effects on symptomatic improvement and on exercise capacity in separate well sized studies.[23,24]

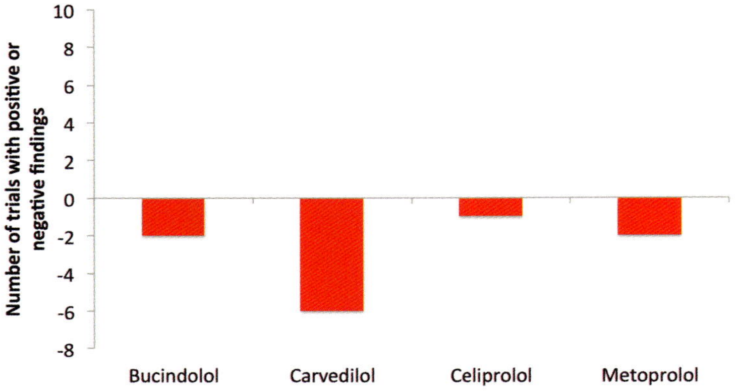

FIGURE 5.3 Overall effect of beta-blockers on exercise capacity in HFrEF[16–24]

Therefore, despite their prognostic benefits beta-blockers do not improve symptoms and functional tolerance in patients with heart failure, but other treatments may do so. Higher doses of beta-blockers are associated with fatigue and with reduced exercise tolerance and therefore it is unlikely that merely increasing the dose of beta-blockade will improve functional capacity in HF patients. Therefore, we may consider down-titration of beta-blocker dose in patients reporting fatigue or a decrease in exercise capacity and replacing this with the alternative heart rate reducing agent, ivabradine that does not decrease (and may actually increase) exercise capacity in HF patients.

Ivabradine

The prognostic benefits of ivabradine in patients with heart failure are coupled with a significant improvement in functional capacity and well-being. In one

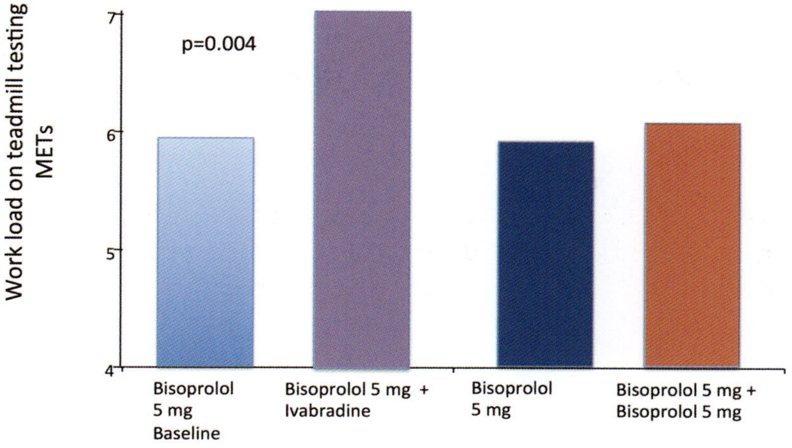

FIGURE 5.4 Ivabradine plus bisoprolol compared to up-titration of bisoprolol on exercise capacity (Amosova et al. ACC. 2010)

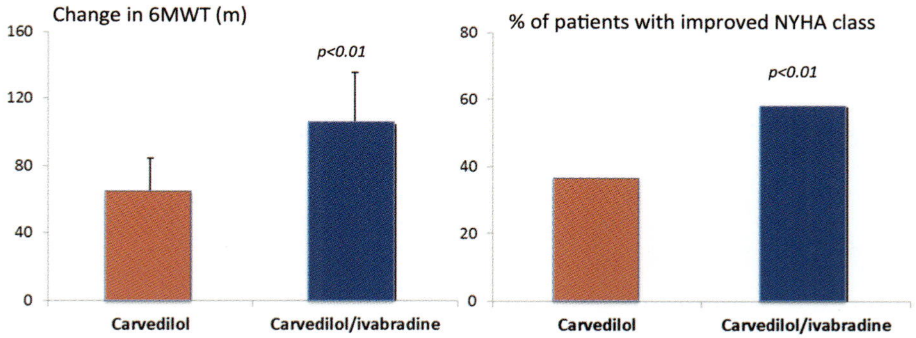

FIGURE 5.5 Ivabradine plus carvedilol compared to uptitration of carvedilol on exercise tolerance and symptoms[23]

early randomised study in patients with underlying coronary artery disease, the combination of ivabradine and bisoprolol was found to be more effective at improving exercise capacity than doubling the bisoprolol dose in patients receiving bisoprolol 5 mg at baseline (Figure 5.4). A further study showed a similar effect with ivabradine added to carvedilol being more effective than uptitrating the dose of cavedilol in patients with HFrEF (Figure 5.5).[23]

In another large randomised study Volterrani et al compared the effect of heart rate reduction with carvedilol, ivabradine, and their combination on exercise capacity in patients with HFrEF receiving maximal dose of ACE inhibitors.[24] The maximal dose of study treatment was more frequently tolerated in patients receiving ivabradine than in those receiving carvedilol. Heart rate was reduced in all three groups, but to a greater extent by combination therapy and the distance walked on the 6-min walking test improved significantly only in patients receiving ivabradine alone or in association with carvedilol while it did not change with carvedilol.(Figure 5.6) The effects observed on the 6MWT were mirrored by similar improvements on MVO_2. Patients receiving ivabradine alone or in combination had better quality of life compared with carvedilol that did not change quality of life compared to baseline values.[24]

The effect of ivabradine on exercise capacity and maximal oxygen consumption was confirmed by another randomised study in patients with ischemic heart failure receiving background beta-blockers. In this study exercise capacity increased doubled and maximal oxygen consumption increased by nearly 30% with ivabradine.[25] These data show that heart rate reduction with ivabradine leads to a better exercise capacity compared to beta blockers alone and that the association of ivabradine with a beta-blocker is effective in improving functional capacity and quality of life compared to beta-blocker alone suggesting that combination therapy is more beneficial than simple beta-blockade. The better effect of ivabradine compared to beta blockers on exercise capacity seems related not only to heart rate reduction, but may also be due to the differing effects of ivabradine and beta-blockers on skeletal muscle perfusion and

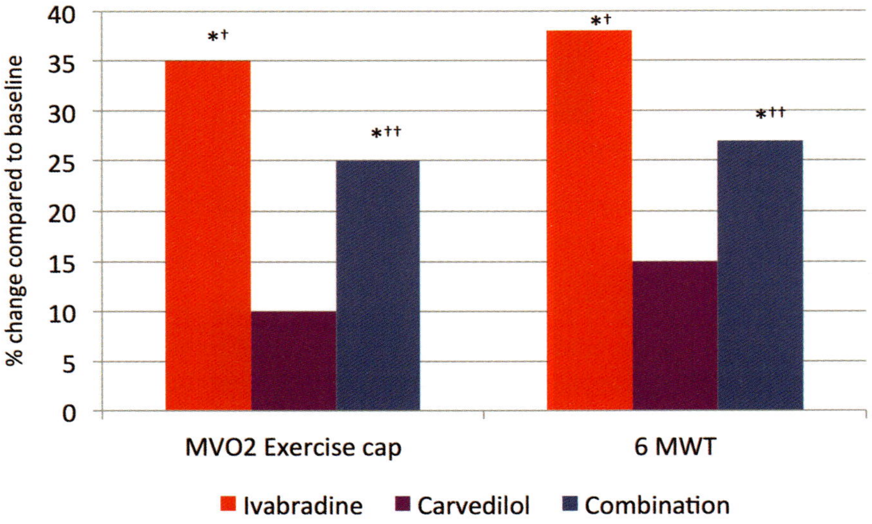

FIGURE 5.6 CARVIVA-HR: Effect of ivabradine carvedilol or combination on exercise capacity.[24] (* $P<0.01$ vs baseline. † $P<0.01$, †† $P<0.02$ vs carvediolol)

performance during exercise. It is well known that beta-blockers impair the alpha-adrenergic-mediated dilation that occurs during exercise while ivabradine preserves the exercise-induced increase in blood flow.[26–28] These effects reflect a better muscle performance during exercise with ivabradine compared to beta-blockers. Given the prognostic effect of ivabradine and its effect on functional capacity and patients related outcomes this drug should always be considered for the treatment of patients with HFrEF. It should always be considered in patients in sinus rhythm. Furthermore, its implementation, associated with an adjustment of the beta-blocker dose, in patients receiving full beta-blockade, especially when reporting fatigue or limited exercise tolerance, may lead to an improved functional status.

ARNI - Angiotensin receptor neprilysin inhibitor

There are no data on the effect of LCZ696 on functional capacity in patients with heart failure. The PARADIGM-HF study showed that the drug was associated with a reduction of the worsening of functional status as assessed by KCCQ change from baseline to month 8. During the first eight months of the study patients receiving LCZ696 had a worsening of the clinical score of –2.99 points compared to –4.63 points in the enalapril group with a significant between-group difference of 1.64 points.[29]

Mineralocorticoid/aldosterone receptor antagonists [MRAs]

While the effect of MRAs on exercise capacity in patients with HFpEF has been extensively investigated, this effect has not been systematically tested in patients with HFrEF. In one randomised study the adjunct of spironolactone to ACEi and diuretics did not increase exercise capacity in HFrEF.[30]

Digoxin and other digitalis glycosides

The effect of digoxin on exercise capacity is neutral. Indeed, only one of four trials showed an improvement in exercise capacity.[31–34] Of importance, the largest of these studies that by itself included more patients than all other studies together (580 patients), did not show any benefit of digoxin on exercise capacity compared to placebo.[35] Whether the effect of digoxin differs between patients in sinus rhythm and those in atrial fibrillation has not been investigated.

Diuretics

Diuretics improve symptoms of congestion in patients with HFrEF.[1] The available data from small trials suggest that in patients with HFrEF conventional diuretics appears to improve exercise capacity when compared to a placebo or to an active comparator. Four trials compared diuretics to active control and showed that diuretics improved exercise capacity in participants.[36–39] Whether the effect of diuretics on exercise capacity was dependent upon the degree of congestion at baseline is not known. All these studies have reported an improvement in symptoms with diuretic therapy.

Metabolic agents

It is well known that altered cardiac metabolism plays an important role in the pathophysiology of heart failure. In particular, chronic HF may be conceived as "a ketosis-prone state" with a switch towards free fatty acid utilisation in the heart. Trimetazidine is an inhibitor of free fatty acid oxidation that shifts cardiac metabolism from free fatty acids to glucose utilisation resulting into a greater production of high-energy phosphates. This translates into a greater myocardial efficiency. Trimetazidine added to standard therapy improves symptoms and exercise capacity in patients with HFrEF of ischaemic and non ischaemic aetiology.

The effect of trimetazidine on symptoms and functional capacity has been tested in several studies in patients with HFrEF. Three meta-analyses of the available data suggest that Trimetazidine improves symptoms, exercise capacity and prognosis in patients with HFrEF.[40–42] The effect of trimetazidine on exercise capacity and symptoms are concordant in all studies and suggest an additive effect on top of medical therapy and on top of cardiac rehabilitation programmes. (Figure 5.7 and 5.8) It has been observed that trimetazidine improves skeletal muscle metabolism.[43–45] This suggests that the main effect of trimetazidine on functional capacity in patients with heart failure may be dependent upon cardiac metabolic effects more than by other mechanisms. Given its positive effect on prognosis in patients with heart failure and its significant effect on symptoms and functional capacity trimetazidine should be always considered in the treatment of patients with heart failure to improve symptoms, quality of life, exercise capacity and prognosis.

Iron supplementation

Iron deficiency occurring in patients with heart failure is associated with impaired functional capacity, poor quality of life, and increased mortality.[46–47]

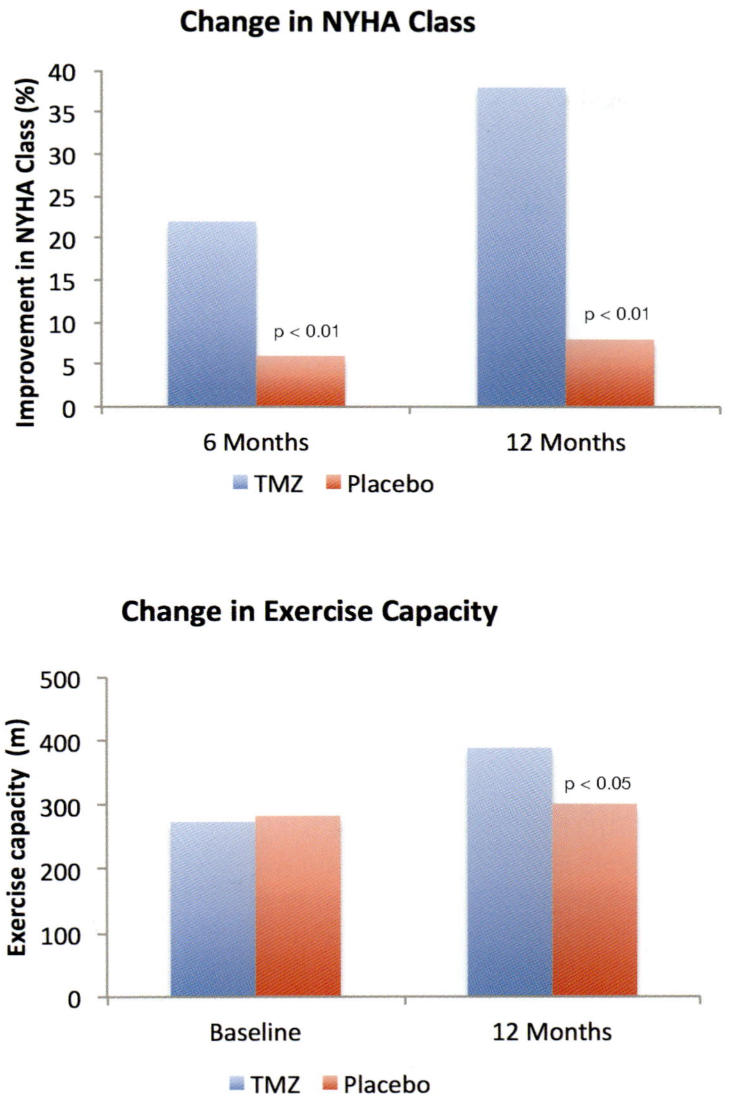

FIGURE 5.7 Effect of trimetazidine in patients with HFrEF (derived from Marazzi G et al. *Eur J Heart Fail.* 2016 (Suppl 1): 51)

The effect of correction of iron deficiency on exercise capacity has been tested in a few clinical studies. The Ferric Iron Sucrose in Heart Failure (FERRIC-HF) study was one of the first placebo-controlled studies that used iron sucrose to replenish iron stores, irrespective of the presence of anaemia. Thirty-seven patients were randomised in a 2 to 1 ratio (either iron sucrose

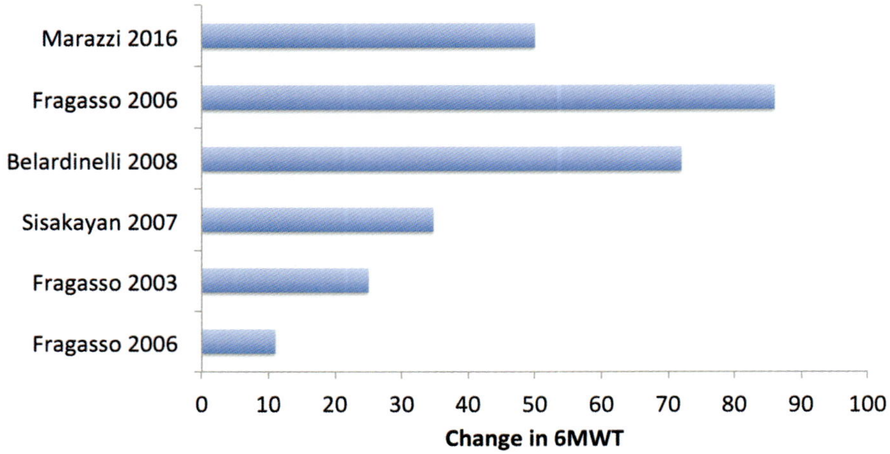

FIGURE 5.8 Effect of trimetazidine on exercise capacity in patients with HFrEF

or placebo) according to their haemoglobin values. Therapy was continued until iron status was normalised. Patients with iron deficiency who received intravenous iron improved their exercise capacity by a mean change in maximal oxygen uptake of almost 2 mL/kg/min.

More recently intravenous administration of ferric carboxymaltose has been consistently shown to improve exercise capacity in patients with HFrEF and low ferritin levels regardless of the presence of anaemia in the FAIR-HF and in the CONFIRM-HF studies (Figure 5.9 and 5.10).[48–49] The FAIR HF study reported a significant improvement with ferric carboxymaltose in the quality of life as measured by the self-reported Patient Global Assessment, improvement (20 metres) in exercise capacity and in the assessment of quality of life measured by the Kansas City Cardiomyopathy Questionnaire (KCCQ).[48] The CONFIRM-HF study showed that ferric carboxymaltose administration in iron-deficient HFrEF patients with and without anaemia caused a sustained improvement in functional capacity over a 12 month period. Of importance patients treated with ferric carboxymaltose showed a significantly reduced risk of hospital admission due to worsening HF during a 1-year follow-up.

A recent meta-analysis of the studies conducted with ferric carboxymaltose in patients with HFrEF with or without anaemia has suggested that this iron formulation reduces re-hospitalisation rates. Therefore, intravenous administration of ferric carboxymaltose is indicated in all patients with HFrEF with ferritin levels <299 μg/l. Oral administration of iron is inadequate to correct low ferritin levels and should not be considered as an alternative to intravenous iron.

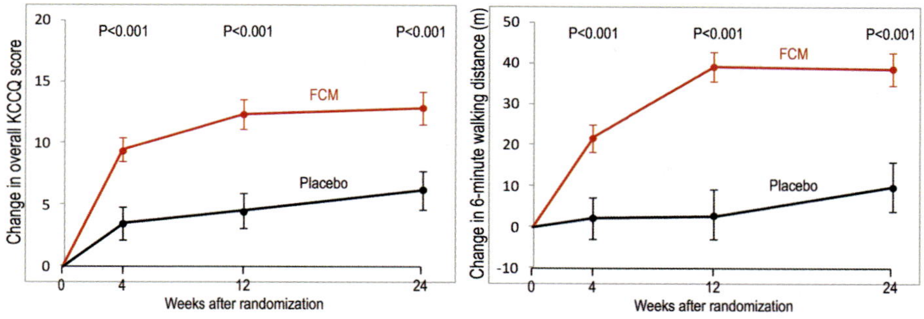

FIGURE 5.9 FAIR-HF change in exercise capacity and KCCQ with ferric carboxymaltose in patients with HFrEF[47]

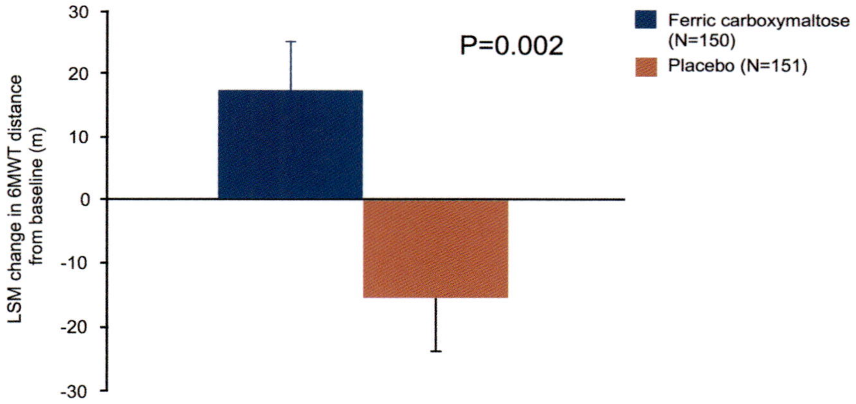

FIGURE 5.10 CONFIRM HF study – change in 6-minutes walking test with ferric carboxymaltose[49]

Testosterone

Testosterone supplementation in patients with HFrEF has been shown to improve exercise capacity regardless of the baseline testosterone levels in both men and women.[50–51] (Figure 5.11) Randomised controlled studies have shown that the effect of testosterone supplementation is related to the improvement in muscle strength and not to any effect on central haemodynamics. A meta-analysis of the available data support the significant benefit of testosterone supplementation in improving exercise capacity in patients with heart failure.[52] The effect is more evident when testosterone supplementation is associated with cardiac rehabilitation programmes. Supra-physiological and supra-therapeutic testosterone supplementation does not have any additional

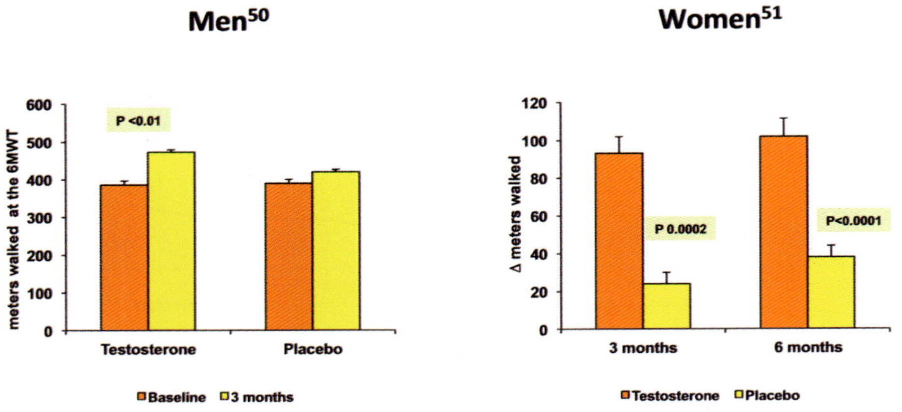

FIGURE 5.11 Effect of testosterone on functional capacity in men and women with HFrEF[50–51]

effect on functional capacity and may worsen clinical status. Testosterone supplementation can be considered in patients with muscle wasting or with cachexia. Supplementation therapy will need adequate monitoring of prostate health and fluid retention.

Calcium channel blockers.

Worsening of heart failure has been reported with all classes of calcium channel blockers. An early small study suggested that amlodipine had a minimal effect on exercise tolerance in heart failure. However, 2 subsequent multicentre studies including patients assessed the effect of amlodipine on exercise capacity and quality of life in patients with HFrEF. Although no statistically significant excess of adverse events were reported the episodes of worsening heart failure were higher in amlodipine-treated patients (10% vs 6.3%). Amlodipine had no effect on exercise tolerance, increasing exercise time less than placebo (53 ± 9 seconds vs 66 ± 9 seconds).[53] Therefore, calcium channel blockers have no effect on exercise tolerance in patients with heart failure. These drugs should not be used in patients with heart failure unless there is a compelling need.

In conclusion, ivabradine, trimetazidine, ferric carboxymaltose and diuretics have consistently shown to improve functional capacity and symptoms in patients with HFrEF because of their effect on long term prognosis these drugs should always be considered in patients with heart failure. Diuretics improve functional capacity and should be prescribed in patients with signs and symptoms of congestions. Cardiac resynchronisation therapy improves functional capacity in patients with HFrEF in whom it is appropriately applied (QRS >130/150 msec according to morphology).

References

1. Ponikowski P, Voors AA, Anker SD, Bueno H, Cleland JG, Coats AJ, Falk V, González-Juanatey JR, Harjola VP, Jankowska EA, Jessup M, Linde C, Nihoyannopoulos P, Parissis JT, Pieske B, Riley JP, Rosano GM, Ruilope LM, Ruschitzka F, Rutten FH, van der Meer P. 2016 ESC Guidelines for the diagnosis and treatment of acute and chronic heart failure: The Task Force for the diagnosis and treatment of acute and chronic heart failure of the European Society of Cardiology (ESC). Developed with the special contribution of the Heart Failure Association (HFA) of the ESC. Eur J Heart Fail. 2016 May 20.
2. Massel D. Ibopamine and survival in severe congestive heart failure: PRIME II. Lancet. 1997 Jul 12; 350(9071): 147.
3. Kamali F, Edwards C. Possible role of metabolite in flosequinan-related mortality. Clin Pharmacokinet. 1995 Dec; 29(6): 396–403.
4. Massie BM, Berk MR, Brozena SC, Elkayam U, Plehn JF, Kukin ML, Packer M, Murphy BE, Neuberg GW, Steingart RM et al. Can further benefit be achieved by adding flosequinan to patients with congestive heart failure who remain symptomatic on diuretic, digoxin, and an angiotensin converting enzyme inhibitor? Results of the flosequinan-ACE inhibitor trial (FACET). Circulation. 1993 Aug; 88(2): 492–501.
5. Packer M, Narahara KA, Elkayam U, Sullivan JM, Pearle DL, Massie BM, Creager MA. Double-blind, placebo-controlled study of the efficacy of flosequinan in patients with chronic heart failure. Principal Investigators of the REFLECT Study. J Am Coll Cardiol. 1993 Jul; 22(1): 65–72.
6. Kuschyk J, Roeger S, Schneider R, Streitner F, Stach K, Rudic B, Weiß C, Schimpf R, Papavasilliu T, Rousso B, Burkhoff D, Borggrefe M. Efficacy and survival in patients with cardiac contractility modulation: long-term single center experience in 81 patients. Int J Cardiol. 2015 Mar 15; 183: 76–81.
7. Giallauria F, Vigorito C, Piepoli MF, Stewart Coats AJ. Effects of cardiac contractility modulation by non-excitatory electrical stimulation on exercise capacity and quality of life: An individual patient's data meta-analysis of randomized controlled trials. Int J Cardiol. 2014 Aug 1; 175(2): 352–7. doi:10.1016/j.ijcard.2014.06.005.
8. Olsson LG, Swedberg K, Clark AL, Witte KK, Cleland JG. Six minute corridor walk test as an outcome measure for the assessment of treatment in randomized, blinded intervention trials of chronic heart failure: a systematic review. Eur Heart J. 2005 Apr; 26(8): 778–93.
9. The Cilazapril-Captopril Multicenter Group. Comparison of the effects of cilazapril and captopril versus placebo on exercise testing in chronic heart failure patients: a double-blind, randomized, multicenter trial. Cardiology. 1995; 86(Suppl. 1): 34–40.
10. Hutcheon SD, Gillespie ND, Crombie IK et al. Perindopril improves six minute walking

distance in older patients with left ventricular systolic dysfunction: a randomized double blind placebo controlled trial. Heart. 2002; 88: 373–377.

11. Granger CB, Ertl G, Kuch J et al. Randomized trial of candesartan cilexetil in the treatment of patients with congestive heart failure and a history of intolerance to angiotensin-converting enzyme inhibitors. Am Heart J. 2000; 139: 609–617.
12. Dickstein K, Chang P, Willenheimer R et al. Comparison of the effects of losartan and enalapril on clinical status and exercise performance in patients with moderate or severe chronic heart failure. J Am Coll Cardiol. 1995; 26: 438–445.
13. Lang RM, Elkayam U, Yellen LG et al. Comparative effects of losartan and enalapril on exercise capacity and clinical status in patients with heart failure. The Losartan Pilot Exercise Study Investigators. J Am Coll Cardiol. 1997; 30: 983–991.
14. McKelvie RS, Yusuf S, Pericak D et al. Comparison of candesartan, enalapril, and their combination in congestive heart failure: randomized evaluation of strategies for left ventricular dysfunction (RESOLVD) pilot study. The RESOLVD Pilot Study Investigators. Circulation. 1999; 100: 1056–1064.
15. Willenheimer R, Helmers C, Pantev E et al. Safety and efficacy of valsartan versus enalapril in heart failure patients. Int J Cardiol. 2002; 85: 261–270.
16. Australia-New Zealand Heart Failure Research Collaborative Group. Effects of carvedilol, a vasodilator-beta-blocker, in patients with congestive heart failure due to ischemic heart disease. Circulation. 1995; 92: 212–218.
17. Australia/New Zealand Heart Failure Research Collaborative Group. Randomized, placebo-controlled trial of carvedilol in patients with congestive heart failure due to ischaemic heart disease. Lancet. 1997; 349: 375–380.
18. Packer M, Colucci WS, Sackner-Bernstein JD et al. Double-blind, placebo-controlled study of the effects of carvedilol in patients with moderate to severe heart failure. The PRECISE Trial. Prospective Randomized Evaluation of Carvedilol on Symptoms and Exercise. Circulation. 1996; 94: 2793–2799.
19. Refsgaard J, Andreasen F, Gotsche O. Divergent outcome between six minute walking test and maximal bicycle test during treatment with carvedilol in patients with mild to moderate heart failure. Eur J Heart Fail. 2000; 2: 95.
20. Krum H, Sackner-Bernstein JD, Goldsmith RL et al. Double-blind, placebo-controlled study of the long-term efficacy of carvedilol in patients with severe chronic heart failure. Circulation. 1995; 92: 1499–1506.
21. Sanderson JE, Chan SK, Yip G et al. Beta-blockade in heart failure: a comparison of carvedilol with metoprolol. J Am Coll Cardiol. 1999; 34: 1522–1528.
22. Metra M, Giubbini R, Nodari S et al. Differential effects of betablockers in patients with heart failure: A prospective, randomized, double-blind comparison of the long-term effects of metoprolol versus carvedilol. Circulation. 2000; 102: 546–551.
23. Bagriy AE, Schukina EV, Samoilova OV, Pricolota OA, Malovichko SI, Pricolota AV, Bagriy EA. Addition of ivabradine to β-blocker improves exercise capacity in systolic heart failure patients in a prospective, open-label study. Adv Ther. 2015 Feb; 32(2): 108–19.
24. Volterrani M, Cice G, Caminiti G, Vitale C, D'Isa S, Perrone Filardi P, Acquistapace F, Marazzi G, Fini M, Rosano GM. Effect of Carvedilol, Ivabradine or their combination

on exercise capacity in patients with Heart Failure (the CARVIVA HF trial). Int J Cardiol. 2011 Sep 1; 151(2): 218–24.
25. Sarullo FM, Fazio G, Puccio D, Fasullo S, Paterna S, Novo S, Di Pasquale P. Impact of "off-label" use of ivabradine on exercise capacity, gas exchange, functional class, quality of life, and neurohormonal modulation in patients with ischemic chronic heart failure. J Cardiovasc Pharmacol Ther. 2010 Dec; 15(4): 349–55.
26. Baumgart D, Haude M, Gorge G et al. Augmented alpha-adrenergic constriction of atherosclerotic human coronary arteries. Circulation. 1999; 99: 2090–7. 568.
27. Heusch G, Baumgart D, Camici P et al. Alpha-adrenergic coronary vasoconstriction and myocardial ischemia in humans. Circulation. 2000; 101: 689–94. 570.
28. Simon L, Ghaleh B, Puybasset L, Giudicelli JF, Berdeaux A. Coronary and hemodynamic effects of S 16257, a new bradycardic agent, in resting and exercising conscious dogs. J Pharmacol Exp Ther. 1995; 275: 659–66.
29. McMurray JJ, Packer M, Desai AS, Gong J, Lefkowitz MP, Rizkala AR, Rouleau JL, Shi VC, Solomon SD, Swedberg K, Zile MR; PARADIGM-HF Investigators and Committees. Angiotensin-neprilysin inhibition versus enalapril in heart failure. N Engl J Med. 2014 Sep 11; 371(11): 993–1004.
30. Kinugawa T, Ogino K, Kato M, Furuse Y, Shimoyama M, Mori M, Endo A, Kato T, Omodani H, Osaki S, Miyakoda H, Hisatome I, Shigemasa C. Effects of spironolactone on exercise capacity and neurohormonal factors in patients with heart failure treated with loop diuretics and angiotensin-converting enzyme inhibitor. Gen Pharmacol. 1998 Jul; 31(1): 93–9.
31. Packer M, Gheorghiade M, Young JB et al. Withdrawal of digoxin from patients with chronic heart failure treated with angiotensin converting-enzyme inhibitors. RADIANCE Study. N Engl J Med. 1993; 329: 1–7.
32. Guyatt GH, Sullivan MJ, Fallen EL et al. A controlled trial of digoxin in congestive heart failure. Am J Cardiol. 1988; 61: 371–375.
33. Uretsky BF, Young JB, Shahidi FE et al. Randomized study assessing the effect of digoxin withdrawal in patients with mild to moderate chronic congestive heart failure: results of the PROVED trial. PROVED Investigative Group. J Am Coll Cardiol. 1993; 22: 955–962.
34. Lader E, Egan D, Hunsberger S et al. The effect of digoxin on the quality of life in patients with heart failure. J Card Fail. 2003; 9: 4–12.
35. Lader E, Egan D, Hunsberger S et al. The effect of digoxin on the quality of life in patients with heart failure. J Card Fail. 2003; 9: 4–12.
36. Boccanelli A, Zachara E, Liberatore SM, Carboni GP, Prati PL. Addition of captopril versus increasing diuretics in moderate but deteriorating heart failure: a double-blind comparative trial. Postgraduate Medical Journal. 1986; 62(Suppl 1): 184–87.
37. Haerer W, Hetzel M, Fehske KL, Fehske KL, Stauch M. The impact of digoxin and diuretics on exercise tolerance in congestive heart failure: a placebo controlled randomised double-blind trial. Circulation. 1989; 80: 1698A.
37. Cowley AJ, Stainer K, Wyne RD, Rowley JM, Hampton JR. Symptomatic assessment of p8tients with heart failure: double-blind comparison of increasing doses of diuretics and captopril in moderate heart failure. Lancet. 1986; 2: 770–72.

39. Richardson A, Bayliss J, Scriven AJ, Sutton GC, Poole-Wilson PA. Double-blind comparison of captopril alone against furosemide plus amiloride in mild heart failure. Lancet. 1987; 2(8561): 709–11.
40. Zhao Y, Peng L, Luo Y, Li S, Zheng Z, Dong R, Zhu J, Liu J. Trimetazidine improves exercise tolerance in patients with ischemic heart disease : A meta-analysis. Herz. 2015 Dec 14. doi:10.1007/s00059-015-4392-2 (epub ahead of print)
41. Zhang L, Lu Y, Jiang H, Zhang L, Sun A, Zou Y, Ge J. Additional use of trimetazidine in patients with chronic heart failure: a meta-analysis. J Am Coll Cardiol. 2012 Mar 6; 59(10): 913–22. doi:10.1016/j.jacc.2011.11.027.
42. Gao D, Ning N, Niu X, Hao G, Meng Z. Trimetazidine: a meta-analysis of randomised controlled trials in heart failure. Heart. 2011 Feb; 97(4): 278–86.
43. Ferraro E, Pin F, Gorini S, Pontecorvo L, Ferri A, Mollace V, Costelli P, Rosano G. Improvement of skeletal muscle performance in ageing by the metabolic modulator Trimetazidine. J Cachexia Sarcopenia Muscle. 2016 Jan 5. Published online 2016 Jan 5. doi:10.1002/jcsm.12097
44. Lopatin YM, Rosano GM, Fragasso G, Lopaschuk GD, Seferovic PM, Gowdak LH, Vinereanu D, Hamid MA, Jourdain P, Ponikowski P. Rationale and benefits of trimetazidine by acting on cardiac metabolism in heart failure. Int J Cardiol. 2016 Jan 15; 203: 909–15.
45. Ferraro E, Giammarioli AM, Caldarola S, Lista P, Feraco A, Tinari A, Salvatore AM, Malorni W, Berghella L, Rosano G. The metabolic modulator trimetazidine triggers autophagy and counteracts stress-induced atrophy in skeletal muscle myotubes. FEBS J. 2013 Oct; 280(20): 5094–5108.
46. Jankowska EA, Rozentryt P, Witkowska A, Nowak J, Hartmann O, Ponikowska B, Borodulin-Nadzieja L, von Haehling S, Doehner W, Banasiak W, Polonski L, Filippatos G, Anker SD, Ponikowski P. Iron deficiency predicts impaired exercise capacity in patients with systolic chronic heart failure. J Card Fail. 2011; 17: 899–906.
47. Jankowska EA, Malyszko J, Ardehali H, Koc-Zorawska E, Banasiak W, von Haehling S, Macdougall IC, Weiss G, McMurray JJ, Anker SD, Gheorghiade M, Ponikowski P. Iron status in patients with chronic heart failure. Eur Heart J. 2013; 34: 827–834.
48. Anker SD, Colet JC, Filippatos G, Willenheimer R, Dickstein K, Drexler H, Lu¨scher TF, Bart B, Banasiak W, Niegowska J, Kirwan BA, Mori C, von Eisenhart Rothe B, Pocock SJ, Poole-Wilson PA, Ponikowski P; for the FAIR-HF Trial Investigators. Ferric carboxymaltose in patients with heart failure and iron deficiency. N Engl J Med. 2009; 361: 2436–2434.
49. Ponikowski P, van Veldhuisen DJ, Comin-Colet J, Ertl G, Komajda M, Mareev V, McDonagh T, Parkhomenko A, Tavazzi L, Levesque V, Mori C, Roubert B, Filippatos G, Ruschitzka F, Anker SD; CONFIRM-HF Investigators. Beneficial effects of long-term intravenous iron therapy with ferric carboxymaltose in patients with symptomatic heart failure and iron deficiency†. Eur Heart J. 2015 Mar 14; 36(11): 657–668.
50. Iellamo F, Volterrani M, Caminiti G, Karam R, Massaro R, Fini M, Collins P, Rosano GM. Testosterone therapy in women with chronic heart failure: a pilot double-blind, randomized, placebo-controlled study. J Am Coll Cardiol. 2010 Oct 12; 56(16): 1310–1316.
51. Caminiti G, Volterrani M, Iellamo F, Marazzi G, Massaro R, Miceli M, Mammi C,

Piepoli M, Fini M, Rosano GM. Effect of long-acting testosterone treatment on functional exercise capacity, skeletal muscle performance, insulin resistance, and baroreflex sensitivity in elderly patients with chronic heart failure a double-blind, placebo-controlled, randomized study. J Am Coll Cardiol. 2009 Sep 1; 54(10): 919–927.

52. Toma M, McAlister FA, Coglianese EE, Vidi V, Vasaiwala S, Bakal JA, Armstrong PW, Ezekowitz JA. Testosterone supplementation in heart failure: a meta-analysis. Circ Heart Fail. 2012 May 1; 5(3): 315–321.
53. Udelson JE, DeAbate CA, Berk M, Neuberg G, Packer M, Vijay NK, Gorwitt J, Smith WB, Kukin ML, LeJemtel T, Levine TB, Konstam MA. Effects of amlodipine on exercise tolerance, quality of life, and left ventricular function in patients with heart failure from left ventricular systolic dysfunction. Am Heart J. 2000 Mar; 139(3): 503–510.

6

Medical treatment of heart failure with reduced ejection fraction – aimed at reducing re-hospitalisations

The prognosis of patients with heart failure has significantly improved in the past decades with the advent of therapies such as angiotensin-converting enzyme (ACE) inhibitors, beta-blockers, mineralocorticoid receptor antagonists (MRAs), ivabradine, LCZ696 and with devices such as implantable cardioverter-defibrillator (ICD) and cardiac resynchronization therapy devices (CRT).[1] By contrast, patients with chronic heart failure that are hospitalised for an episode of de-compensation continue have a high mortality and excessive hospital readmission rates.[2]

Hospitalisations for heart failure are frequent in treatment-naïve patients as well as in patients with chronic heart failure and in those who had been recently hospitalised because of a recent episode of de-compensation. High rates of re-hospitalisation are more frequent in patients with co-morbidities and in those with advanced heart failure.[2] It is estimated that nearly 50% of patients with heart failure will be re-hospitalised within 6 months of discharge, and that 70% of these re-hospitalisations are related to worsening of their heart failure.[3]

Precipitating factors for a new hospitalisation episode in patients with heart failure include cardiac factors such as myocardial ischaemia, new onset or rapid rate atrial fibrillation, and un-controlled hypertension.[4] However, a sizeable proportion of hospitalisations occurring in patients with heart failure are non-cardiac or precipitated by extra-cardiac factors, such as exacerbations of COPD, infections and anaemia or by patient-related factors, such as medication non-adherence, use of non-steroidal anti-inflammatory drugs and the effects of drug-drug interactions.[5]

Therefore, heart failure hospitalisations are relevant causes of poor prognosis and quality of life in patients with heart failure. Hospital admissions are extremely distressing for patients, especially the older ones and they are heralds of an accelerated disease progression. They are also the major driver of the economic burden of heart failure. Consequently, treatments that may positively reduce hospitalisation rates have a significant effect on quality of life, disease progression and the costs of care.

Predicting heart failure readmission

Several studies have suggested different predictors for re-hospitalisation in patients with HFrEF but, given the different models of health care (mostly private in US, mostly national health services in Europe, mixed models elsewhere), it is difficult to develop a risk model that may adequately predict the risk of readmission.

Pathophysiological indices of heart failure severity may predict higher rehospitalisation rates. Some of these indices are related to elevated filling pressures, such as jugular venous pressure, orthopnoea, echocardiographic filling patterns and plasma levels of cardiac biomarkers such as natriuretic peptides and cardiac troponins.[1,5] Inadequate diuretic dosing or intolerance of neuro-hormonal antagonists because of hypotension or renal dysfunction are also likely indicators of de-compensation requiring re-hospitalisation. Both cardiac and non cardiac co-morbidities (atrial fibrillation, ischaemic heart disease, chronic kidney disease, diabetes mellitus, anaemia, pulmonary disease) also increase the risk for heart failure hospitalisations.[1]

Heart failure hospitalisations are higher in patients with psychosocial and/or socioeconomic factors that limit adherence and treatment compliance while high adherence to guidelines implemented through disease management programs reduces re-admission rates.[6] Therefore, evidence based therapies and international guidelines should be implemented during the in-patient and out-patient settings at all stages of the disease in patients with heart failure.

Disease management programs

These programs are a multidisciplinary, integrated approach to disease management that include different forms of patient care ranging from direct patient follow-up (outpatient clinic or at home) or remote support such as by telephone calls or telemonitoring. The DIAL trial[7] that randomly assigned 1,518 patients with heart failure to either routine care or an intervention with an explanatory booklet and periodic telephone calls by a nurse enforcing self-management resulted in a lower rates of heart failure hospitalisations (26.3% vs 31%) at a mean follow up of 16 months. A Dutch study including 1,023 patients with HF assigned to a control group with regular cardiologist follow up and 2 interventions with either additional basic support or intensive support by a nurse found no differences in mortality or heart failure re-hospitalisations amongst the 3 groups.[8]

A systematic review[9] of 29 randomised controlled studies of multidisciplinary disease management programmes conducted either in a clinic or a non-clinic setting showed reduced mortality (RR 0.75, 95% CI 0.59–0.96), heart failure hospitalisations (RR 0.74, 95% CI 0.63–0.87), and all-cause hospitalizations (RR 0.81, 95% CI 0.71–0.92). Similarly programmes aimed at enhancing patient self-care activities reduced HF hospitalizations (RR 0.66, 95% CI 0.52–0.83) and all-cause hospitalizations (RR 0.73, 95% CI 0.57–0.93) but had no effect on mortality (RR 1.14, 95% CI 0.57–1.94).

Telemonitoring is used to communicate with patients and obtain health status and physiologic data (weight, ECG, fluid status etc.) remotely. A meta-analysis of 14 randomised studies suggested that remote monitoring programmes could reduce the rates of admission to hospital for chronic heart failure by 21% (95% confidence interval 11% to 31%) and all cause mortality by 20% (8% to 31%) in patients with heart failure.[10] More recently, recent large randomised controlled studies using tele-monitoring or usual care yielded

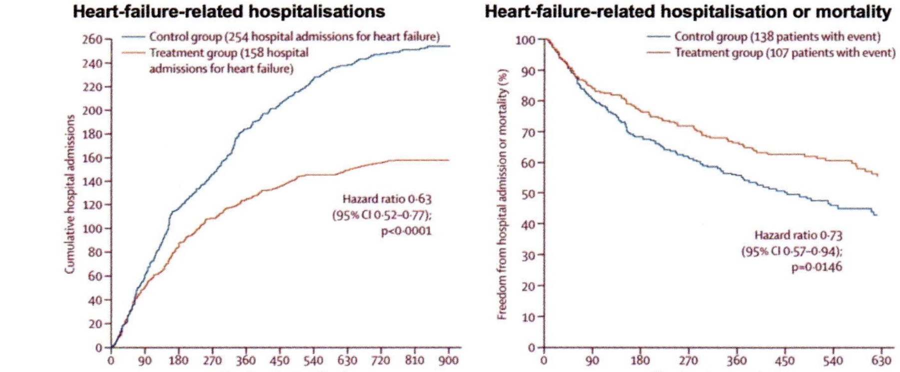

FIGURE 6.1 CHAMPION study – wireless pulmonary artery haemodynamic monitoring with CardioMEMS in heart failure

conflicting results suggesting that tele-monitoring should be tailored to the local healthcare settings.[11,12]

On the other hand, a disease management program with therapies adjusted according to physiological signals of pulmonary artery pressures measured directly with the implantable CardioMEMS Heart Sensor has been shown to reduce by 39% heart failure hospitalizations in the CHAMPION trial.[6] (see Figure 6.1) Furthermore, a cost-effectiveness analysis showed that integrating CardioMEMS wireless pulmonary artery pressure monitoring into the management of heart failure patients is a cost effective addition to the heart failure treatment pathway in appropriate patients.

Medical therapy aimed at reducing hospitalisations

Management of fluid overload

Prevention of clinical and subclinical congestion with adequate use of diuretics reduces re-hospitalisation rates.[1] Loop diuretic therapy is the mainstay of congestion management. Metolazone, a long-acting thiazide-like diuretic, may be used in those patients who are poorly responsive to loop diuretics but it is associated with a significant risk of hyponatraemia especially if used chronically.[2]

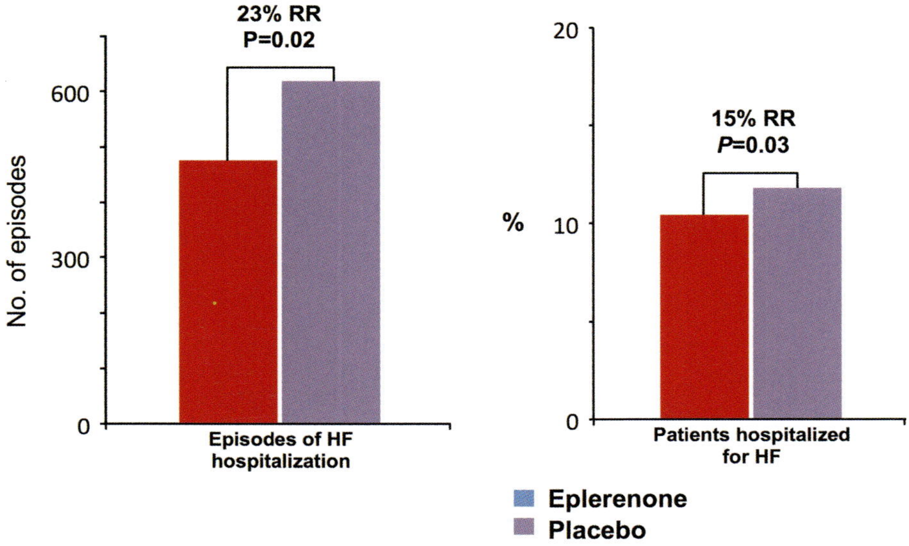

FIGURE 6.2 EPHESUS study – Effect of eplerenone on heart failure hospitalizations. From Pitt B et al, *N Engl J Med.* 2003; 348: 1309–1321

Its pulsed use has less effect on plasma sodium levels. Mineralocorticoid receptor antagonists are particularly useful in controlling fluid balance and modulating the neuro-humoral balance. Spironolactone and eplerenone both significantly reduce (35%) re-hospitalization rates and are indicated in all patients with heart failure.[1] (see Figure 6.2)

In patients with fluid retention presenting with hyponatraemia, and/or impaired renal function, the vasopressin antagonist tolvaptan should be considered although it has no effect on long term prognosis and re-hospitalisation rates.[13]

Renin-angiotensin-aldosterone system inhibitors (RAASi)

RAASi including angiotensin-converting enzyme (ACE) inhibitors, angiotensin receptor blockers (ARBs), and aldosterone receptor antagonists (ARAs), reduce the risk for mortality and hospitalization in patients with existing HF.[1] After the CONSENSUS study (COoperative North Scandinavian ENalapril SUrvival Study),[14] several trials with angiotensin-converting enzyme (ACE) inhibitors, including captopril, lisinopril, ramipril, and trandolapril, confirmed the benefit of in different clinical settings, including asymptomatic left ventricular dysfunction and post-infarction heart failure.[15] ARBs have also been investigated in chronic heart failure and have been shown to reduce re-hospitalisation rates. However, given that the benefit of ARBs is sensibly less than that of ACEi they should only be used in patients who are intolerant to ACEi.[1]

A meta-analysis of the large randomised controlled trials has demonstrated that RAASi reduce the risk of re-hospitalisation by 20% and that this effect is independent by the degree of left ventricular dysfunction.[16] (Figure 6.3) However, the proportional effects on all end points decreased with increasing mean left ventricular ejection fraction. These findings support the indication for use of an ACEi and a MRA in all patients with HFrEF with a class IA recommendation.

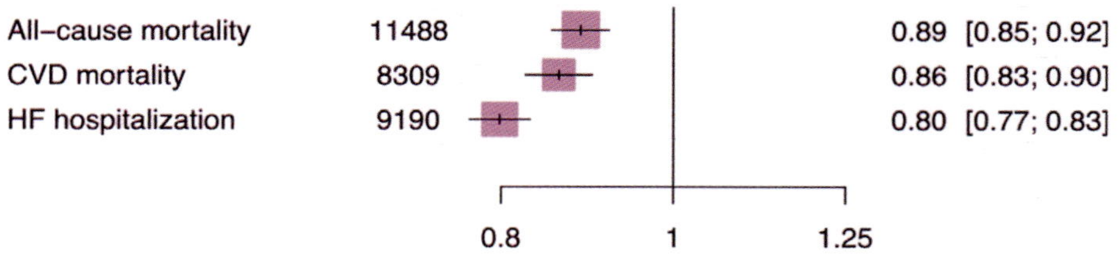

FIGURE 6.3 Effect of RAASi on all cause mortality, cardiovascular mortality and hospitalisation for heart failure.[16]

Beta-blockers

The use of beta-blockers has been demonstrated to prevent deterioration of myocardial function, and to improve prognosis in patients with HFrEF because of their effect on the inhibition of neuro-hormonal activation. Several studies and meta-analyses have demonstrated that the prognostic benefit of beta-blockers depends on the degree of heart rate reduction rather than on the administered dose.[17]

Systematic reviews of the randomised trials of beta blockers in heart failure have shown a beneficial effects on mortality and hospital admissions but only in patients in sinus rhythm.[18] A recent individual patient meta-analysis of 18,254 patients included in all the adequately sized randomised studies testing the effect of beta-blockers in patients with HFrEF has shown that the prognostic benefit of beta-blockers observed in patients in sinus rhythm in not seen in patients with atrial fibrillation. This meta-analysis has also shown a consistent benefit of β blockers versus placebo for hospital admission outcomes in patients with sinus rhythm while a significantly attenuated effect in those with atrial fibrillation (HR 0.78 vs 0.91 sinus rhythm vs atrial fibrillation, p<005). Therefore, beta-blockers reduce events and hospitalisations in patients with HFrEF in sinus rhythm while in those in atrial fibrillation the extent of the benefit of beta-blockers is less clear. In patients with atrial fibrillation, however, beta-blockers are still indicated inferring their benefit from the studies conducted mostly in patients HFrEF and in sinus rhythm.

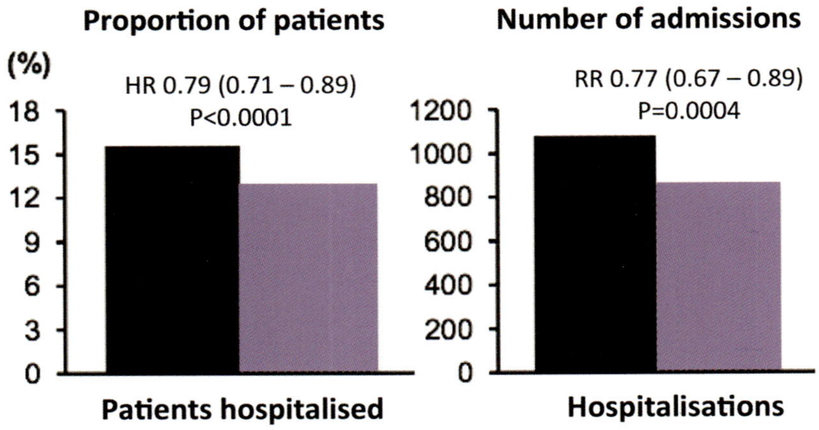

FIGURE 6.4 PARADIGM HF – Effect of LCZ696 on heart failure hospitalisations.[19]

Angiotensin II Receptor Neprilysin Inhibitor

The PARADIGM HF study has shown that LCZ696 is superior to Enalapril in reducing mortality and morbidity in patients with heart failure and elevated natriuretic peptide levels.[19] Further to the mortality benefit, LCZ696 significantly reduced the rate of hospitalisation for heart failure compared to enalapril (hazard ratio, 0.79; 95% CI, 0.71–0.89; P<0.001). LCZ696 also reduced the rates of hospitalisations for a cardiovascular reason (hazard ratio, 0.88; 95% CI, 0.81–0.95; P<0.001) or for any reason (hazard ratio, 0.88; 95% CI, 0.82–0.94; P<0.001). (Figure 6.4) Therefore, LCZ696 is indicated for all patients with HFrEF with symptomatic heart failure despite treatment with an ACEi (or an ARB). In this case the treatment with ACEi or ARB should be discontinued at least 36 hours before the first dose of LCZ696.

Ivabradine

In patients with stable heart failure with a heart rate above 70 beats per minute (bpm) included in the SHIFT trial (Systolic Heart failure treatment with the If inhibitor ivabradine Trial), heart rate was associated with an increased risk of cardiovascular death and heart failure hospitalizations, which translates into a 3% increase in risk for every 1-bpm increase from baseline heart rate and 15% increase in risk for every 5-bpm increase.[20]

Heart rate reduction with ivabradine reduced the composite outcome of cardiovascular death and heart failure hospitalisation in patients with HFrEF

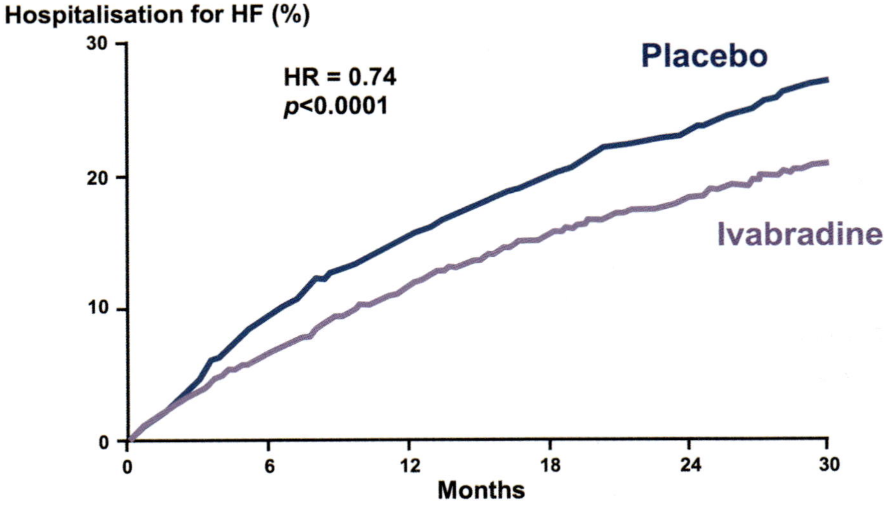

FIGURE 6.5 SHIFT study – Effect of ivabradine on heart failure hospitalisations.[21]

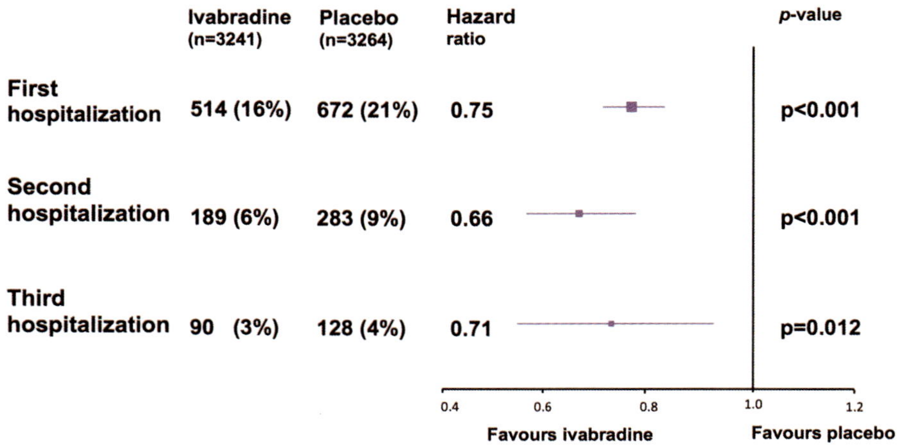

FIGURE 6.6 SHIFT study effect of ivabradine on heart failure hospitalisation.[21]

with a heart rate above 70 bpm and cardiovascular death and total mortality in the subgroup of patients with a heart rate above 75 bpm.[21] Hospitalisations for heart failure were reduced by 26% with ivabradine, the effect appeared early and was constant throughout the study. (Figure 6.5)

Furthermore the SHIFT study showed amongst the 1,186 patients a 34% reduction in second heart failure hospitalizations among those who were admitted once and a 29% reduction among those who were admitted twice.[21] (Figure 6.6) All-cause and cardiovascular hospitalisations were similarly reduced by ivabradine and, in patients with more than one admission, ivabradine prolonged the time to a second admission with a longer time out of hospital free of worsening heart failure. Indeed, the time from one admission to the subsequent one was prolonged by 17% by ivabradine and significantly fewer patients with HFrEF who received ivabradine during the study suffered a second hospital admission.[21]

Despite a sizeable proportion of patients included in the SHIFT trial receiving MRAs, ivabradine had a highly significant effect on outcomes, including hospitalisations for heart failure, independent of the effect of MRAs.

The SHIFT study also showed that ivabradine is effective in preventing early re-admission in patients with HFrEF who had been hospitalised for heart failure. Indeed, among those patients who suffered a first hospitalization during the study, patients receiving ivabradine had a reduced occurrence of re-hospitalisation in the following 30 days compared to those receiving placebo (IRR 0.70, $p<0.05$).[21] These findings clearly show the benefit of ivabradine, on a background of beta-blockade, angiotensin-converting enzyme inhibitors, mineralocorticoid receptor antagonists, and diuretics in reducing early and later re-hospitalisations for heart failure.

After discharge from heart failure hospitalization, under-treatment of patients with β-blockers and angiotensin-converting enzyme (ACE) inhibitors occurs often in patients with low blood pressure. A proportion ranging between 15% to 25% of patients discharged from hospital for an episode of decompensation have low blood pressure (ie, <120 mm Hg), which reduces the possibility to fully implement medical therapy and puts them at an increased risk for poor outcomes. The combination of higher heart rates and low blood pressure further increases event rates in patients with heart failure. In this population of patients with heart failure ivabradine showed a consistent effect on the reduction of hospitalisations and events.[16,17] Therefore, an early initiation of ivabradine, which is not accompanied by blood pressure reduction, leads to a higher proportion of patients receiving evidence-based treatment in the year after discharge as recently shown.

Digitalis

The DIG (Digitalis Investigators Group) trial suggested that digoxin, when added to diuretics and ACE inhibitors in patients with chronic HF in sinus rhythm, decreases hospitalizations without adversely affecting survival.[22] However, in DIG trial the effect of digoxin on the reduction of heart failure hospitalisations was offset by a significant increase of other cardiovascular hospitalizations (hazard ratio: 1.20; 95% confidence interval: 1.05 to 1.38).

More recently an analysis of de novo use of digoxin in adults with incident systolic heart failure included in the database of the Kaiser Permanente Northern California system showed that digoxin use was associated not only with higher rates of death (14.2 vs. 11.3 per 100 person-years) but also with higher rates of heart failure hospitalization (28.2 vs. 24.4 per 100 person-years) than non-use.[23] Therefore, digoxin has not consistently shown to reduce re-hospitalisations and its use should be limited to selected patients as outlined in other chapters.[1]

The reduction in re-hospitalisation for heart failure is an important therapeutic goal in patients with heart failure, because of the effect of hospitalisations on well-being and prognosis. LCZ696 and ivabradine have been shown not only to reduce events in patients with HFrEF but also to reduce heart failure hospitalisations occurring both as first events, and as recurrent hospitalisations with a similar degree of efficacy. Given the neutral effect of ivabradine on blood pressure, this drug should be always considered in patients in sinus rhythm. LCZ696 has some blood pressure lowering effect that may limit its implementation in some patients. Therefore, in order to fully benefit from the prognostic benefits of these two drugs patients who are still symptomatic after the administration of an ACEi a beta-blocker and a MRA should be switched to these therapies and controlling heart rate with the combination of beta-blockers and ivabradine. Treatments should be implemented with appropriate disease management programs and fluid retention should be monitored with devices like the CardioMEMS that have been proven to effectively reduce events.

References

1. Ponikowski P, Voors AA, Anker SD, Bueno H, Cleland JG, Coats AJ, Falk V, González-Juanatey JR, Harjola VP, Jankowska EA, Jessup M, Linde C, Nihoyannopoulos P, Parissis JT, Pieske B, Riley JP, Rosano GM, Ruilope LM, Ruschitzka F, Rutten FH, van der Meer P. 2016 ESC Guidelines for the diagnosis and treatment of acute and chronic heart failure: The Task Force for the diagnosis and treatment of acute and chronic heart failure of the European Society of Cardiology (ESC). Developed with the special contribution of the Heart Failure Association (HFA) of the ESC. Eur J Heart Fail. 2016 May 20.
2. Maggioni AP, Dahlstro¨m U, Filippatos G, Chioncel O, Leiro MC, Drozdz J, Fruhwald F, Gullestad L, Logeart D, Fabbri G, Urso R, Metra M, Parissis J, Persson H, Ponikowski P, Rauchhaus M, Voors AA, Nielsen OW, Zannad F, Tavazzi L, Crespo Leiro M, Drozdz J, Fruhwald F, Gullestad L, Logeart D, Fabbri G, Urso R, Metra M, Parissis J, Persson H, Ponikowski P, Rauchhaus M, Voors AA, Nielsen OW, Zannad F, Tavazzi L. EURObservational Research Programme: regional differences and 1-year follow-up results of the Heart Failure Pilot Survey (ESC-HF Pilot). Eur J Heart Fail 2013; 15: 808–817.
3. Ross JS, Chen J, Lin Z, Bueno H, Curtis JP, Keenan PS, Normand SL, Schreiner G, Spertus JA, Vidan MT, Wang Y, Wang Y, Krumholz HM. Recent national trends in readmission rates after heart failure hospitalization. Circulation. 2010; 3: 97–103.
4. Gheorghiade M, Abraham WT, Albert NM, Greenberg BH, O'Connor CM, She L, Stough WG, Yancy CW, Young JB, Fonarow GC. Systolic blood pressure at admission, clinical characteristics, and outcomes in patients hospitalized with acute heart failure. JAMA. 2006; 296: 2217–2226.
5. Gheorghiade M, Vaduganathan M, Fonarow GC, Bonow RO. Rehospitalization for Heart Failure Problems and Perspectives. J Am Coll Cardiol 2013; 61: 391–403.
6. Abraham WT, Adamson PB, Bourge RC, Aaron MF, Costanzo MR, Stevenson LW, Strickland W, Neelagaru S, Raval N, Krueger S, Weiner S, Shavelle D, Jeffries B, Yadav JS. Wireless pulmonary artery haemodynamic monitoring in chronic heart failure: a randomised controlled trial. Lancet. 2011; 377: 658–666.
7. GESICA Investigators. Randomised trial of telephone intervention in chronic heart failure: DIAL trial. BMJ. 2005 Aug 20; 331(7514): 425.
8. Jaarsma T, van der Wal MH, Lesman-Leegte I, Luttik ML, Hogenhuis J, Veeger NJ, Sanderman R, Hoes AW, van Gilst WH, Lok DJ, Dunselman PH, Tijssen JG, Hillege HL, van Veldhuisen DJ; Coordinating Study Evaluating Outcomes of Advising and Counseling in Heart Failure (COACH) Investigators. Effect of moderate or intensive

disease management program on outcome in patients with heart failure: Coordinating Study Evaluating Outcomes of Advising and Counseling in Heart Failure (COACH). Arch Intern Med. 2008 Feb 11; 168(3): 316–24.

9. McAlister FA, Stewart S, Ferrua S, McMurray JJ. Multidisciplinary strategies for the management of heart failure patients at high risk for admission: a systematic review of randomized trials. J Am Coll Cardiol. 2004 Aug 18; 44(4): 810–9.
10. Clark RA, Inglis SC, McAlister FA, Cleland JG, Stewart S. Telemonitoring or structured telephone support programmes for patients with chronic heart failure: systematic review and meta-analysis. BMJ. 2007 May 5; 334(7600): 942.
11. Hindricks G, Taborsky M, Glikson M, Heinrich U, Schumacher B, Katz A, Brachmann J, Lewalter T, Goette A, Block M, Kautzner J, Sack S, Husser D, Piorkowski C, Søgaard P; IN-TIME study group. Implant-based multiparameter telemonitoring of patients with heart failure (IN-TIME): a randomised controlled trial. Lancet. 2014 Aug 16; 384(9943): 583–90.
12. Boyne JJ, Vrijhoef HJ, Crijns HJ, De Weerd G, Kragten J, Gorgels AP; TEHAF investigators. Tailored telemonitoring in patients with heart failure: results of a multicentre randomized controlled trial. Eur J Heart Fail. 2012 Jul; 14(7): 791–801.
13. O'Connor CM, Miller AB, Blair JE, et al. Causes of death and rehospitalization in patients hospitalized with worsening heart failure and reduced left ventricular ejection fraction: results from Efficacy of Vasopressin Antagonism in Heart Failure Outcome Study with Tolvaptan (EVEREST) program. Am Heart J 2010; 159: 841–9.
14. The Consensus Trial Study Group. Effects of enalapril on mortality in severe congestive heart failure. N Engl J Med.1987; 316: 1429–1435.
15. López-Sendón J, Swedberg K, McMurray J, et al. Expert consensus document on angiotensin converting enzyme inhibitors in cardiovascular disease. The Task Force on ACE-inhibitors of the European Society of Cardiology. Eur Heart J. 2004; 25: 1454–1470.
16. Emdin CA, Callender T, Cao J, McMurray JJV, Rahimi K. Meta-Analysis of Large-Scale Randomized Trials to Determine the Effectiveness of Inhibition of the Renin-Angiotensin Aldosterone System in Heart Failure. Am J Cardiol 2015; 116: 155e161.
17. McAlister FA ; Wiebe N ; Ezekowitz JA ; Leung AA ; Armstrong PW. Meta-analysis: beta-blocker dose, heart rate reduction, and death in patients with heart failure. Ann Intern Med 2009 Jun 2; Vol. 150 (11), pp. 784–94.
18. Kotecha D, Holmes J, Krum H, Altman DG, Manzano L, Cleland JGF, Lip GYH, Coats AJS, Andersson B, Kirchhof P, von Lueder TG, Wedel H, Rosano G, Shibata MC, Rigby A, Flather MD. Efficacy of b blockers in patients with heart failure plus atrial fibrillation: an individual-patient data meta-analysis. Lancet 2014; 384: 2235–2243.
19. McMurray JJ, Packer M, Desai AS, Gong J, Lefkowitz MP, Rizkala AR, Rouleau JL, Shi VC, Solomon SD, Swedberg K, Zile MR; PARADIGM-HF Investigators and Committees. Angiotensin-neprilysin inhibition versus enalapril in heart failure. N Engl J Med. 2014 Sep 11; 371(11): 993–1004.
20. Swedberg K, Komajda M, Böhm M, et al. Ivabradine and outcomes in chronic heart failure (SHIFT): a randomised placebo-controlled study. Lancet 2010; 376: 875–85.
21. Borer JS, Böhm M, Ford I, et al. Effect of ivabradine on recurrent hospitalization for

worsening heart failure in patients with chronic systolic heart failure: the SHIFT study. Eur Heart J 2012; 33: 2813–20.
22. The Digitalis Investigation Group. The effect of digoxin on mortality and morbidity in patients with heart failure. N Engl J Med 1997; 336: 525–33.
23. Freeman JV, Yang J, Sung SH, et al. Effectiveness and safety of digoxin among contemporary adults with incident systolic heart failure. Circ Cardiovasc Qual Outcomes 2013; 6: 525–33.

7

Approach to the treatment of heart failure with preserved ejection fraction and mid-range ejection fraction

Introduction

In this chapter, treatment of heart failure (HF) with preserved ejection fraction (HFpEF) and of HF with mid-range ejection fraction (HFmrEF) according to the recent European Society of Cardiology (ESC) guidelines[1] will be described. Since clinical trials on HFpEF have included also patients with HFmrEF, due to the lack of a consensual definition (see Chapter 1), ESC recommendations here described apply to both phenotypes. As a consequence of the recent characterisation of this HF syndrome, it is expected that upcoming research will provide data specifically regarding HFmrEF and tailored recommendations will be developed.

Symptomatic treatment of HFpEF/HFmrEF

Patients with HFpEF and HFmrEF are often treated with diuretics, beta-blockers, MRAs and ACEIs or ARBs in clinical trials,[2] similarly to patients with HFrEF. This may be possibly due to an anecdotal clinical assumption that these drugs may be beneficial in HFpEF/HFmrEF patients. Other reasons may be the lack of adherence to the guidelines and the treatment of comorbidities.[1] However, so far, the efficacy of these agents on mortality or morbidity in patients with HFpEF/HFmrEF has not been clearly demonstrated. Thus, the ESC guidelines indicate as the goal of therapy in HFpEF/HFmrEF the relief of symptomatology and the consequential improvement in quality of life.[3] In fact, patients in these categories are often elderly and present worse symptomatology, more comorbidities and poorer prognosis than HFrEF patients.[4,1]

In order to alleviate symptoms/signs, the ESC guidelines recommend the use of diuretics to improve congestion in HFpEF/HFmrEF patients. Congestion improvement has been obtained in HF patients regardless of the degree of left ventricular ejection fraction impairment.[5] Conversely, there is the need to investigate whether relief of symptoms/signs may be obtained with beta-blockers and MRAs in HFpEF/HFmrEF. There are inconsistencies about the efficacy of ARBs in HFpEF.[6–7] As for ACEIs, the Perindopril in elderly people with chronic heart failure (PEP-CHF) trial[8] has found that perindropil improved symptoms and exercise capacity with also fewer HF hospitalisations. Further studies are awaited to draw firm conclusions.

For hospitalisation reduction, the following agents have been found to be efficacious in HFpEF patients: nebivolol,[9–11] digoxin,[12] spironolactone[13] and candesartan.[6] It must be remembered that these findings are secondary analyses and therefore not as firm as primary end-point analyses of major RCTs. Notably, nebivolol has been shown its efficacy on a combined endpoint of death or cardiovascular hospitalization[9,11] in older patients with HFrEF, HFpEF and HFmrEF. These conclusions apply for patients in sinus rhythm. In HFpEF patients with atrial fibrillation, there is no evidence on digoxin, inconsistent results for ARBs or ACEIs and data so far collected suggest beta-blockers to be inefficacious.[1]

Finally, exercise capacity is compromised in HFpEF/HFmrEF and is often associated with an increased blood pressure response to exercise and chronotropic inability. Exercise training has been shown to improve exercise tolerance and to be safe[14,4] and is therefore indicated by the ESC guidelines.

Treatment of comorbidities in HFpEF/HFmrEF

In the clinical management of HFpEF/HFmrEF patients, assessment and treatment of comorbidities are pivotal. The guidelines recommend screening in these patients for both cardiovascular and non-cardiovascular comorbidities. In case the patient presents comorbidities, these should be treated with safe and effective interventions. This should facilitate improved symptoms, quality of life and/or prognosis. Patients with HFpEF/HFmrEF and atrial fibrillation should receive an anticoagulant to reduce the risk of thromboembolic events, according to the ESC guidelines (see also Chapter 13). It should be noted that antiplatelet agents are not effective and NOACs are not indicated in the case of renal dysfunction due to the haemorrhagic risk.[1] The guidelines also indicate to consider rate control in these patients with caution. To date, due to the paucity of studies, it is unknown which agent should be chosen for rate-control and whether ablation strategies should be applied.

Another comorbidity that often affects HFpEF/HFmrEF patients is myocardial ischaemia, which also impacts symptomatology and prognosis. Further studies are needed to clarify whether revascularization has efficacy on symptoms, morbidity or mortality in HFpEF/HFmrEF. According to the ESC guidelines, HFpEF/HFmrEF patients with angina should be treated following the same protocol as HFrEF patients.[15] Also, HFpEF/HFmrEF patients may benefit from the treatment of hypertension, especially systolic hyptertension.[16,17] Whereas beta-blockers are not effective in reducing systolic blood pressure, diuretics, ACEIs, ARBs and MRAs may be efficacious.[1] Circumstantial evidence[18] suggests that HFpEF/HFmrEF patients with hypertension should not be treated with an ARB in combination with ACEIs and beta-blockers.

Hyperglycaemia may be treated with metformin, the preferred oral agent in HFpEF patients according to the ESC Guidelines on diabetes.[19] Empagliflozin has been found[20] to decrease blood pressure and body weight, possibly acting on glycosuria and osmotic diuresis and this may in part explain the significant reduction in HF related hospitalisations it produced (see Chapter 13). However, an aggressive treatment of dysglycaemia should be avoided as it may be unsafe.[21,22]

What treatments can be indicated for the new concept of HFmrEF?

Treatment of HFmrEF remains largely empirical as no acknowledged standards currently exist. However, clinical trials on HFpEF published so far may give some indications to the clinician treating a patient with HFmrEF, although upcoming studies specifically including patients with this diagnosis are strongly needed. Clinical trials with upper left ventricular ejection fraction boundaries above 40% have yielded conclusions that may be clinically useful for the symptomatic treatment of HFmrEF patients. The Study of the Effects of Nebivolol Intervention on Outcomes and Hospitalisation in Seniors with Heart Failure (SENIORS)[9,10] suggests that nebivolol is well tolerated and effective in patients with HF, even when left ventricular systolic function is not markedly depressed. In this trial, nebivolol reduced the composite outcome of all-cause mortality or cardiovascular hospital admissions in older patients with HF[10] and nebivolol treatment was associated with a one-third reduction in the risk of ischaemic events, independently of ejection fraction.[23]

Similarly, regardless of ejection fraction, digoxin reduced mortality and hospitalisations in a wide spectrum of ambulatory chronic HF patients in the Digitalis Investigation Group: Preserved Ejection Fraction (DIG-PEF) trial.[12] Digoxin may be considered to alleviate HF symptoms before considering aggressive therapy (i.e. with high-dose non-potassium-sparing diuretics)[12] that may increase mortality and hospitalisations[24] in HFmrEF patients.

Results from clinical trials with RAAS antagonists need to be interpreted with caution, for both HFpEF and HFmrEF. The Treatment of preserved cardiac function heart failure with an Aldosterone antagonist (TOPCAT)[13] failed to show improvement in mortality with the use of spironolactone in HFpEF. However, as aforementioned, there is some evidence on RAAS efficacy on morbidity in HFpEF. Perindopril showed improvement in exercise capacity, and candesartan decreased hospitalisations for HF; however, irbesartan showed no benefit in either improving quality of life or decreasing hospitalisations for HF.[25] Thus, data collected so far suggest therapy with RAAS antagonists for HFpEF/HFmrEF only in presence of comorbidities such as hypertension, diabetes mellitus, or coronary artery disease.[25,26]

References:

1. Ponikowski, P., A. A. Voors, S. D. Anker, H. Bueno, J. Cleland, A. Coats, V. Falk, J. R. Gonzalez-Juanatey, V. Harjola, E. Jankowska, M. Jessup, C. Linde, P. Nihoyannopoulos, J. T. Parissis, B. Pieske, J. Riley, G. M. C. Rosano, L. Ruilope, F. Ruschitzka, F. H. Rutten and P. van der Meer (2016). 2016 ESC Guidelines for the diagnosis and treatment of acute and chronic heart failure. European Heart Journal.
2. Maggioni, A. P., S. D. Anker, U. Dahlstrom, G. Filippatos, P. Ponikowski, F. Zannad, O. Amir, O. Chioncel, M. C. Leiro, J. Drozdz, A. Erglis, E. Fazlibegovic, C. Fonseca, F. Fruhwald, P. Gatzov, E. Goncalvesova, M. Hassanein, J. Hradec, A. Kavoliuniene, M. Lainscak, D. Logeart, B. Merkely, M. Metra, H. Persson, P. Seferovic, A. Temizhan, D. Tousoulis, L. Tavazzi and E. S. C. Heart Failure Association of the (2013). Are hospitalized or ambulatory patients with heart failure treated in accordance with European Society of Cardiology guidelines? Evidence from 12,440 patients of the ESC Heart Failure Long-Term Registry. Eur J Heart Fail 15(10): 1173–1184.
3. Lewis, E. F., G. A. Lamas, E. O'Meara, C. B. Granger, M. E. Dunlap, R. S. McKelvie, J. L. Probstfield, J. B. Young, E. L. Michelson, K. Halling, J. Carlsson, B. Olofsson, J. J. McMurray, S. Yusuf, K. Swedberg, M. A. Pfeffer and C. Investigators (2007). Characterization of health-related quality of life in heart failure patients with preserved versus low ejection fraction in CHARM. Eur J Heart Fail 9(1): 83–91.
4. Fukuta, H., T. Goto, K. Wakami and N. Ohte (2016). Effects of drug and exercise intervention on functional capacity and quality of life in heart failure with preserved ejection fraction: A meta-analysis of randomized controlled trials. Eur J Prev Cardiol 23(1): 78–85.

5. Faris, R., M. Flather, H. Purcell, M. Henein, P. Poole-Wilson and A. Coats (2002). Current evidence supporting the role of diuretics in heart failure: a meta analysis of randomised controlled trials. Int J Cardiol 82(2): 149–158.
6. Yusuf, S., M. A. Pfeffer, K. Swedberg, C. B. Granger, P. Held, J. J. McMurray, E. L. Michelson, B. Olofsson, J. Ostergren, C. Investigators and Committees (2003). Effects of candesartan in patients with chronic heart failure and preserved left-ventricular ejection fraction: the CHARM-Preserved Trial. Lancet 362(9386): 777–781.
7. Massie, B. M., P. E. Carson, J. J. McMurray, M. Komajda, R. McKelvie, M. R. Zile, S. Anderson, M. Donovan, E. Iverson, C. Staiger, A. Ptaszynska and I. P. Investigators (2008). Irbesartan in patients with heart failure and preserved ejection fraction. N Engl J Med 359(23): 2456–2467.
8. Cleland, J. G., M. Tendera, J. Adamus, N. Freemantle, L. Polonski, J. Taylor and P.-C. Investigators (2006). The perindopril in elderly people with chronic heart failure (PEP-CHF) study. Eur Heart J 27(19): 2338–2345.
9. Flather, M. D., M. C. Shibata, A. J. Coats, D. J. Van Veldhuisen, A. Parkhomenko, J. Borbola, A. Cohen-Solal, D. Dumitrascu, R. Ferrari, P. Lechat, J. Soler-Soler, L. Tavazzi, L. Spinarova, J. Toman, M. Bohm, S. D. Anker, S. G. Thompson, P. A. Poole-Wilson and S. Investigators (2005). Randomized trial to determine the effect of nebivolol on mortality and cardiovascular hospital admission in elderly patients with heart failure (SENIORS). Eur Heart J 26(3): 215–225.
10. van Veldhuisen, D. J., A. Cohen-Solal, M. Bohm, S. D. Anker, D. Babalis, M. Roughton, A. J. Coats, P. A. Poole-Wilson, M. D. Flather and S. Investigators (2009). Beta-blockade with nebivolol in elderly heart failure patients with impaired and preserved left ventricular ejection fraction: Data From SENIORS (Study of Effects of Nebivolol Intervention on Outcomes and Rehospitalization in Seniors With Heart Failure). J Am Coll Cardiol 53(23): 2150–2158.
11. Mulder, B. A., D. J. van Veldhuisen, H. J. Crijns, M. Bohm, A. Cohen-Solal, D. Babalis, M. Roughton, M. D. Flather, A. J. Coats and I. C. Van Gelder (2012). Effect of nebivolol on outcome in elderly patients with heart failure and atrial fibrillation: insights from SENIORS. Eur J Heart Fail 14(10): 1171–1178.
12. Ahmed, A., M. W. Rich, J. L. Fleg, M. R. Zile, J. B. Young, D. W. Kitzman, T. E. Love, W. S. Aronow, K. F. Adams, Jr. and M. Gheorghiade (2006). Effects of digoxin on morbidity and mortality in diastolic heart failure: the ancillary digitalis investigation group trial. Circulation 114(5): 397–403.
13. Pitt, B., M. A. Pfeffer, S. F. Assmann, R. Boineau, I. S. Anand, B. Claggett, N. Clausell, A. S. Desai, R. Diaz, J. L. Fleg, I. Gordeev, B. Harty, J. F. Heitner, C. T. Kenwood, E. F. Lewis, E. O'Meara, J. L. Probstfield, T. Shaburishvili, S. J. Shah, S. D. Solomon, N. K. Sweitzer, S. Yang, S. M. McKinlay and T. Investigators (2014). Spironolactone for heart failure with preserved ejection fraction. N Engl J Med 370(15): 1383–1392.
14. Edelmann, F., G. Gelbrich, H. D. Dungen, S. Frohling, R. Wachter, R. Stahrenberg, L. Binder, A. Topper, D. J. Lashki, S. Schwarz, C. Herrmann-Lingen, M. Loffler, G. Hasenfuss, M. Halle and B. Pieske (2011). Exercise training improves exercise capacity and diastolic function in patients with heart failure with preserved ejection fraction: results of the Ex-DHF (Exercise training in Diastolic Heart Failure) pilot study. J Am Coll Cardiol 58(17): 1780–1791.

15. Windecker, S., P. Kolh, F. Alfonso, J. P. Collet, J. Cremer, V. Falk, G. Filippatos, C. Hamm, S. J. Head, P. Juni, A. P. Kappetein, A. Kastrati, J. Knuuti, U. Landmesser, G. Laufer, F. J. Neumann, D. J. Richter, P. Schauerte, M. Sousa Uva, G. G. Stefanini, D. P. Taggart, L. Torracca, M. Valgimigli, W. Wijns and A. Witkowski (2015). 2014 ESC/EACTS guidelines on myocardial revascularization. EuroIntervention 10(9): 1024–1094.
16. Beckett, N. S., R. Peters, A. E. Fletcher, J. A. Staessen, L. Liu, D. Dumitrascu, V. Stoyanovsky, R. L. Antikainen, Y. Nikitin, C. Anderson, A. Belhani, F. Forette, C. Rajkumar, L. Thijs, W. Banya, C. J. Bulpitt and H. S. Group (2008). Treatment of hypertension in patients 80 years of age or older. N Engl J Med 358(18): 1887–1898.
17. Mancia, G., R. Fagard, K. Narkiewicz, J. Redon, A. Zanchetti, M. Bohm, T. Christiaens, R. Cifkova, G. De Backer, A. Dominiczak, M. Galderisi, D. E. Grobbee, T. Jaarsma, P. Kirchhof, S. E. Kjeldsen, S. Laurent, A. J. Manolis, P. M. Nilsson, L. M. Ruilope, R. E. Schmieder, P. A. Sirnes, P. Sleight, M. Viigimaa, B. Waeber, F. Zannad and M. Task Force (2013). 2013 ESH/ESC Guidelines for the management of arterial hypertension: the Task Force for the management of arterial hypertension of the European Society of Hypertension (ESH) and of the European Society of Cardiology (ESC). J Hypertens 31(7): 1281–1357.
18. Sakata, Y., K. Nochioka, M. Miura, T. Takada, S. Tadaki, S. Miyata, N. Shiba and H. Shimokawa (2013). Supplemental benefit of an angiotensin receptor blocker in hypertensive patients with stable heart failure using olmesartan (SUPPORT) trial – rationale and design. J Cardiol 62(1): 31–36.
19. Ryden, L., E. Standl, M. Bartnik, G. et al. (2007). Guidelines on diabetes, pre-diabetes, and cardiovascular diseases: executive summary. The Task Force on Diabetes and Cardiovascular Diseases of the European Society of Cardiology (ESC) and of the European Association for the Study of Diabetes (EASD). Eur Heart J 28(1): 88–136.
20. Zinman, B., C. Wanner, J. M. Lachin, D. Fitchett, E. Bluhmki, S. Hantel, M. Mattheus, T. Devins, O. E. Johansen, H. J. Woerle, U. C. Broedl, S. E. Inzucchi and E.-R. O. Investigators (2015). Empagliflozin, Cardiovascular Outcomes, and Mortality in Type 2 Diabetes. N Engl J Med 373(22): 2117–2128.
21. Gilbert, R. E. and H. Krum (2015). Heart failure in diabetes: effects of anti-hyperglycaemic drug therapy. Lancet 385(9982): 2107–2117.
22. Udell, J. A., M. A. Cavender, D. L. Bhatt, S. Chatterjee, M. E. Farkouh and B. M. Scirica (2015). Glucose-lowering drugs or strategies and cardiovascular outcomes in patients with or at risk for type 2 diabetes: a meta-analysis of randomised controlled trials. Lancet Diabetes Endocrinol 3(5): 356–366.
23. Ambrosio, G., M. D. Flather, M. Bohm, A. Cohen-Solal, A. Murrone, F. Mascagni, G. Spinucci, M. G. Conti, D. J. van Veldhuisen, L. Tavazzi and A. J. Coats (2011). beta-blockade with nebivolol for prevention of acute ischaemic events in elderly patients with heart failure. Heart 97(3): 209–214.
24. Domanski, M., J. Norman, B. Pitt, M. Haigney, S. Hanlon, E. Peyster and D. Studies of Left Ventricular (2003). Diuretic use, progressive heart failure, and death in patients in the Studies Of Left Ventricular Dysfunction (SOLVD). J Am Coll Cardiol 42(4): 705–708.
25. Oghlakian, G. O., I. Sipahi and J. C. Fang (2011). Treatment of heart failure with

preserved ejection fraction: have we been pursuing the wrong paradigm? Mayo Clin Proc 86(6): 531–539.

26. Senni, M., W. J. Paulus, A. Gavazzi, A. G. Fraser, J. Diez, S. D. Solomon, O. A. Smiseth, M. Guazzi, C. S. Lam, A. P. Maggioni, C. Tschope, M. Metra, S. L. Hummel, F. Edelmann, G. Ambrosio, A. J. Stewart Coats, G. S. Filippatos, M. Gheorghiade, S. D. Anker, D. Levy, M. A. Pfeffer, W. G. Stough and B. M. Pieske (2014). New strategies for heart failure with preserved ejection fraction: the importance of targeted therapies for heart failure phenotypes. Eur Heart J 35(40): 2797–2815.

8

Treatment of patients in the vulnerable phase (at discharge or early after discharge)

Introduction

The clinical course of heart failure (HF) includes a period in which the patient is at increased risk of death or rehospitalisation for HF. This period is termed the "vulnerable phase"[1] and occurs during the peri-acute HF phase, due to microenvironmental changes in the cardiovascular system.[2] Typically, the vulnerability phase starts from the onset of an acute HF event leading to admission, continues through a peri-discharge period and lasts up to 6 months after discharge.[2,3] These poor post-discharge outcomes also represent a significant socioeconomic burden.[4]

Patient vulnerability occurs regardless of the type of acute episode, but the individual impact may vary.[2] Although the exact mechanisms leading to readmissions are not fully clarified and there are many possible precipitants of rehospitalisation for HF,[5] the following factors have been identified and may be controlled: persistent congestion, end-organ damage and comorbidities.[6] Despite the increased risk for adverse outcomes, the vulnerability phase may also represent a window of opportunity[7] because in those who survive this period successfully, with the assistance of appropriate management, a phase of long-term stability can be expected.[2]

The vulnerable phase may be seen as a continuum[8] but it is usually divided into three periods that may be overlapping: a very early phase, an early phase, and a late phase. Each period has its own prioritised therapeutic goals[8] based on the patient's clinical characteristics (Table 8.1).

TABLE 8.1 The vulnerability phase in HF patients

Definition	Timing and clinical characteristics	Management indications
Very early vulnerable sub-phase	From the acute episode up to a few days post discharge. Patient is often discharged before complete relief of congestion.	Patient should be discharged when haemodynamically stable, euvolaemic, and managed on stable long-term oral medication, with stable organ function and once provided with a tailored education and advice plan about self-care. ACEi should be implemented at full dose and diuretics should be adjusted in order to maintain euvolaemia.
Early vulnerable sub-phase	After the discharge of a relatively well-decongested patient.	Beta-blockers should be implemented with caution. Ivabradine can be easily implemented in therapy and together with beta-blockers helps in controlling heart rate to target.
Late vulnerable sub-phase	Typically extends up to 6 months. Watch for possible beginnings of haemodynamic congestion before overt systemic congestion.	Continue multidisciplinary management programmes designed to improve outcomes through structured follow-up and monitoring. Optimisation of medical treatment.

ACEi = angiotensin-converting enzyme inhibitors; HF = heart failure

Very early vulnerability sub-phase

The risk of rehospitalisations is particularly high in the period that immediately follows the acute episode.[2] Thus, early recognition of this vulnerability state and the implementation of management strategies are pivotal to successful navigation of this high-risk phase. The desired management plan should be therefore conceived before discharge[9] to provide clinical stabilisation, relief of symptoms, recovery of and protection from end-organ damage and to reduce the risk of complications.[8] In this phase, the accurate identification of signs of haemodynamic congestion is a priority because congestion leads to high vulnerability and an especially poor prognosis.[10] Patients should be discharged when they have been haemodynamically stable for at least 24–48 hours,[10] euvolaemic, stabilised on long-term oral medication, and when they have stable organ function, including that of the kidney and liver in particular.[2]

Unfortunately often pre-existing therapy has been discontinued or reduced during the acute hospitalisation and this must be taken into account as a prognostic risk factor for subsequent readmissions and death. In severe, acutely decompensated HF patients previously on long-term beta-blocker therapy discontinuing the therapy has been found to lead to a worse prognosis.[11] On the contrary, the continuation of pre-existing beta-blocker therapy at admission has been found to predict the best prognosis.[11]

According to the 2016 European Society of Cardiology (ESC) guidelines,[9] acute HF patients should be discharged when clinical parameters are stable and after an individualised educational programme about self-care has been implemented (see below). Once congestion is stabilised and, if possible, euvolemia is re-established, the use of ACEi's (or if not tolerated an ARB) is indicated. Specifically, the guidelines recommend ACEi's (or an ARB) in patients with HFrEF to improve symptoms and exercise capacity, reduce the risk of HF hospitalisation and increase survival.[9] Such a therapy should be preferably initiated before discharge. The discharge plan should be formulated also taking into account the level of HF-related biomarkers, in particular the measurement of natriuretic peptides (NPs) and cardiac troponins (see Chapter 3).

The aetiology is an important factor to take into account. It has been demonstrated that rehospitalisations are more likely to occur in patients with ischaemic HF[12] and the risk of subsequent episodes of ischaemia needing active management may be better assessed by measuring levels of NPs and troponins before discharge. The use of biomarker-directed therapy adjustment has been shown significantly to reduce HF events and, also, to be cost-saving.[13]

For all these reasons, a multidisciplinary approach is the recommended strategy for the management of the vulnerable patient (see below). Pre- and post-discharge management should follow the standards of care developed by the Heart Failure Association (HFA) of the ESC.[14] Finally, according to the guidelines, patients should be visited by their general practitioner within 1 week of discharge. The hospital cardiology team should follow up the patients within 2 weeks of discharge, if possible.

Early vulnerability sub-phase

In this period, occurring after the patient has been decongested, and is euvolaemic, the ESC guidelines[9] recommend to continue the disease management plan individually designed to prevent rehospitalisations, and to improve symptoms, survival and quality of life. Due to neuroendocrine activation, elevated heart rate and low blood pressure may appear in this phase.[15] Of note, an elevated heart rate is associated with an increased risk of cardiovascular death and hospitalisations for HF.[16]

If heart rate is still high despite therapy with beta-blockers, the addition of ivabradine is the best approach, also to improve HF-related symptoms and well-being.[17] A recent randomised study[18] found that the early co-administration of ivabradine and beta-blockers (24 hours after hospital admission) was more efficacious and safer in acute patients hospitalised with HFrEF in reducing heart rate after hospital discharge, than treatment with beta-blockers alone. Also, a significant improvement in the ejection fraction was observed, consistent with data from the Systolic Heart failure treatment with the If inhibitor ivabradine Trial (SHIFT) study.[15] Finally, a significant decrease in BNP values and a trend toward a reduction in advanced functional classes were observed in the combined therapy group. Thus, the addition of ivabradine to beta-blockers may be introduced earlier than previously indicated by the SHIFT trial (i.e. ≥4 weeks after hospitalisation) to achieve heart rate control and improve prognosis.

Late vulnerability sub-phase

This vulnerability period may last up to 6 months after discharge and is related to late reactivation of the renin-angiotensin-aldosterone system (RAAS). The aim of management in this late phase is to lead the vulnerable patient to a subsequent phase of stability. As haemodynamic congestion may appear before overt systemic congestion, diuretics should be adjusted in order to maintain euvolaemia long-term. A gradual rise in ventricular filling pressures may be observed in patients prior to, and predicting, subsequent overt congestion. Thus, other HF episodes might well occur and should be prevented by the above-described multidisciplinary assessment of clinical symptoms/signs and biomarkers.[13]

Poor prognosis in the late phase could be prevented by adequate up-titration of ACEI (or ARB), beta-blockers, MRAs, and ivabradine following the current ESC guidelines.[9] Optimisation of disease modifying therapies, such as device therapy, should be also ensured.[2]

To improve prognosis, the management plan should also consists of an *educational programme* with appropriate lifestyle adjustments, as recommended by the guidelines. Indeed, education leads to an improvement in patient skills of self-care after discharge.[19,20] Such "self-empowerment" is in line with the prospective of a continuous, "at-a-distance" care[21] that may be obtained through *telemedicine*, another component of the management plan. This term indicates a comprehensive approach that includes structured telephone support, remote distance monitoring of biomarkers (e.g. weight, heart rate, blood pressure, etc) and the use of implantable devices.[7,21,22] There is also evidence that telemedicine may improve outcomes and reduce HF hospitalisations.[23]

The recommendations from ESC guidelines[9] for multidisciplinary

TABLE 8.2 Multidisciplinary management and monitoring of patients with HF according to the ESC guidelines

Recommendation	Class
It is recommended that regular aerobic exercise is encouraged in patients with HF to improve functional capacity and symptoms.	I
It is recommended that regular aerobic exercise is encouraged in stable patients with HFrEF to reduce the risk of HF hospitalisation.	I
It is recommended that patients with HF are enrolled in a multidisciplinary care management programme to reduce the risk of HF hospitalisation and mortality.	I
Referral to primary care for long-term follow-up may be considered for stable patients with HF who are on optimal therapy to monitor for effectiveness of treatment, disease progression and patient adherence.	IIb
Monitoring of pulmonary artery pressures using a wireless implantable haemodynamic monitoring system (CardioMems) may be considered in symptomatic patients with HF with previous HF hospitalisation in order to reduce the risk of recurrent HF hospitalisation.	IIb
Multiparameter monitoring based on ICD (IN-TIME approach) may be considered in symptomatic patients with HFrEF (LVEF $\leq$ 35%) in order to improve clinical outcomes.	IIb

Class of recommendation: I = evidence and/or general agreement that a given treatment or procedure is beneficial, useful, effective; II = conflicting evidence and/or a divergence of opinion about the usefulness/efficacy of the given treatment or procedure (IIa: weight of evidence/opinion is in favor of usefulness/efficacy; IIb: usefulness/efficacy is less well established by evidence/opinion); III: evidence or general agreement that the given treatment or procedure is not useful/effective, and in some cases may be harmful.

HF = heart failure; ICD = implantable cardioverter-defibrillator; IN-TIME = Implant-based multiparameter telemonitoring of patients with heart failure; HFrEF = heart failure with reduced ejection fraction; LVEF = left ventricular ejection fraction.

management and monitoring of patients with HF are listed in Table 8.2. Other components of the management plan for HF patients according to ESC guidelines are listed in Box 8.1.

In conclusion, HF adverse outcomes should be prevented by using a combination of strategies[24] that may lead the vulnerable patient to a stability phase. It is pivotal that patients are monitored by a multi-professional HF service[9] and evidence-based guideline recommendations such as those from the ESC/HFA should be followed.

BOX 8.1 Components of management programmes for patients with HF according to the ESC guidelines

- Optimised medical and device management
- Adequate patient education, with special emphasis on adherence and self-care
- Patient involvement in symptom monitoring and flexible diuretic use
- Follow-up after discharge (regular clinic and/or home-based visits; possibly telephone support or remote monitoring)
- Increased access to healthcare (through in-person follow-up and by telephone contact; possibly through remote monitoring)
- Facilitated access to care during episodes of decompensation
- Assessment of (and appropriate intervention in response to) an unexplained change in weight, nutritional status, functional status, quality of life, or laboratory findings
- Access to advanced treatment options
- Provision of psychosocial support to patients and family and/or caregivers

ESC = European Society of Cardiology; HF = heart failure.

References:

1. Gheorghiade, M., P. S. Pang, A. P. Ambrosy, G. Lan, P. Schmidt, G. Filippatos, M. Konstam, K. Swedberg, T. Cook, B. Traver, A. Maggioni, J. Burnett, L. Grinfeld, J. Udelson and F. Zannad (2012). A comprehensive, longitudinal description of the in-hospital and post-discharge clinical, laboratory, and neurohormonal course of patients with heart failure who die or are re-hospitalized within 90 days: analysis from the EVEREST trial. Heart Fail Rev 17(3): 485–509.
2. Yilmaz, M. B. and A. Mebazaa (2015). Definition and characteristics of the vulnerable phase in heart failure. Medicographia 37(2): 1–5.
3. Follath, F., M. B. Yilmaz, J. F. Delgado, J. T. Parissis, R. Porcher, E. Gayat, N. Burrows, A. McLean, F. Vilas-Boas and A. Mebazaa (2011). Clinical presentation, management and outcomes in the Acute Heart Failure Global Survey of Standard Treatment (ALARM-HF). Intensive Care Med 37(4): 619–626.
4. Farmakis, D., G. Filippatos, J. Parissis and J. Lekakis (2015). The social and economic burden of hospitalization for heart failure. Medicographia 37(2): 135–138.
5. Gheorghiade, M., M. Vaduganathan, G. C. Fonarow and R. O. Bonow (2013). Rehospitalization for heart failure: problems and perspectives. J Am Coll Cardiol 61(4): 391–403.
6. Metra, M., V. Carubelli, I. Castrini, A. Ravera, E. Sciatti and C. Lombardi (2015). Postdischarge outcomes of patients hospitalized for heart failure. Medicographia 37(2): 139–143.

7. Zamorano, J. L. and V. C. Lozano (2015). Impact of quality improvement initiatives in patients hospitalized for heart failure. Medicographia 37(2): 163–169.
8. Ponikowski, P. and E. A. Jankowska (2015). Treatment optimization in heart failure patients from admission to discharge. Medicographia 37(2): 149–154.
9. Ponikowski, P., A. A. Voors, S. D. Anker, H. Bueno, J. Cleland, A. Coats, V. Falk, J. R. Gonzalez-Juanatey, V. Harjola, E. Jankowska, M. Jessup, C. Linde, P. Nihoyannopoulos, J. T. Parissis, B. Pieske, J. Riley, G. M. C. Rosano, L. Ruilope, F. Ruschitzka, F. H. Rutten and P. van der Meer (2016). 2016 ESC Guidelines for the diagnosis and treatment of acute and chronic heart failure. European Heart Journal.
10. Gheorghiade, M., F. Follath, P. Ponikowski, J. H. Barsuk, J. E. Blair, J. G. Cleland, K. Dickstein, M. H. Drazner, G. C. Fonarow, T. Jaarsma, G. Jondeau, J. L. Sendon, A. Mebazaa, M. Metra, M. Nieminen, P. S. Pang, P. Seferovic, L. W. Stevenson, D. J. van Veldhuisen, F. Zannad, S. D. Anker, A. Rhodes, J. J. McMurray, G. Filippatos, C. European Society of and M. European Society of Intensive Care (2010). Assessing and grading congestion in acute heart failure: a scientific statement from the acute heart failure committee of the heart failure association of the European Society of Cardiology and endorsed by the European Society of Intensive Care Medicine. Eur J Heart Fail 12(5): 423–433.
11. Bohm, M., A. Link, D. Cai, M. S. Nieminen, G. S. Filippatos, R. Salem, A. Cohen Solal, B. Huang, R. J. Padley, M. Kivikko and A. Mebazaa (2011). Beneficial association of beta-blocker therapy on recovery from severe acute heart failure treatment: data from the Survival of Patients With Acute Heart Failure in Need of Intravenous Inotropic Support trial. Crit Care Med 39(5): 940–944.
12. Chun, S., J. V. Tu, H. C. Wijeysundera, P. C. Austin, X. Wang, D. Levy and D. S. Lee (2012). Lifetime analysis of hospitalizations and survival of patients newly admitted with heart failure. Circ Heart Fail 5(4): 414–421.
13. Bocchi, E. A., D. A. Brito, O. Chioncel, A. Fong, M. Hülsmann, E. A. Jankowska, M. Loutfi, A. Lupi, Y. F. M. Nosir, E. B. Reyes, S. N. Tereschenko, M. B. Yilmaz and B. Yoo (2015). Can biomarkers guide the assessment and management of heart failure patients after discharge from hospitals? Medicographia 37(2): 171–184.
14. Mebazaa, A., M. B. Yilmaz, P. Levy, P. Ponikowski, W. F. Peacock, S. Laribi, A. D. Ristic, E. Lambrinou, J. Masip, J. P. Riley, T. McDonagh, C. Mueller, C. deFilippi, V. P. Harjola, H. Thiele, M. F. Piepoli, M. Metra, A. Maggioni, J. J. McMurray, K. Dickstein, K. Damman, P. M. Seferovic, F. Ruschitzka, A. F. Leite-Moreira, A. Bellou, S. D. Anker and G. Filippatos (2015). Recommendations on pre-hospital and early hospital management of acute heart failure: a consensus paper from the Heart Failure Association of the European Society of Cardiology, the European Society of Emergency Medicine and the Society of Academic Emergency Medicine – short version. Eur Heart J 36(30): 1958–1966.
15. Böhm, M. (2015). Challenges in predicting heart failure readmission: focus on heart rate. Medicographia 37(2): 197–201.
16. Bohm, M., K. Swedberg, M. Komajda, J. S. Borer, I. Ford, A. Dubost-Brama, G. Lerebours, L. Tavazzi and S. Investigators (2010). Heart rate as a risk factor in chronic heart failure (SHIFT): the association between heart rate and outcomes in a randomised placebo-controlled trial. Lancet 376(9744): 886–894.

17. Elyubaeva, I. (2015). Procoralan: new opportunities for vulnerable heart failure patients. Medicographia 37(2): 185–192.
18. Hidalgo, F. J., M. Anguita, J. C. Castillo, S. Rodriguez, L. Pardo, E. Duran, J. J. Sanchez, C. Ferreiro, M. Pan, D. Mesa, M. Delgado and M. Ruiz (2016). Effect of early treatment with ivabradine combined with beta-blockers versus beta-blockers alone in patients hospitalised with heart failure and reduced left ventricular ejection fraction (ETHIC-AHF): A randomised study. Int J Cardiol 217: 7–11.
19. Cowie, M. R. (2015). Postdischarge assessment and management of patients with heart failure. Medicographia 37(2): 155–162.
20. Jourdain, P. (2015). Therapeutic education: which tool for whom? Medicographia 37(2): 193–196.
21. Zugck, C. (2015). Telemonitoring in heart failure management: what is needed to make it fit for routine use? Medicographia 37(2): 202–207.
22. Komajda, M. (2015). Hospitalization for heart failure: can we prevent it? Can we predict it? Medicographia 37(2): 119–124.
23. Inglis, S. C., R. A. Clark, F. A. McAlister, S. Stewart and J. G. Cleland (2011). Which components of heart failure programmes are effective? A systematic review and meta-analysis of the outcomes of structured telephone support or telemonitoring as the primary component of chronic heart failure management in 8323 patients: Abridged Cochrane Review. Eur J Heart Fail 13(9): 1028–1040.
24. López-Sendón, J. and N. Montoro (2015). The changing landscape of heart failure outcomes. Medicographia 37(2): 125–134.

9

Implantable cardioverter-defibrillators and cardiac resynchronization therapy in the treatment of heart failure with reduced ejection fraction

Introduction

It has been long acknowledged that electrical-conduction disturbances may be both a cause of heart failure and a consequence of it.[1,2] In fact, many patients with heart failure have an asynchronous contraction pattern of the heart muscle that further reduces the heart ability to pump blood.[3] Electrical disturbances may therefore result in progressive left ventricular dysfunction, due to the added effects of HF-related electrical dyssynchrony.[4] For this reason, device therapy may play a key role in the management of patients with heart failure and reduced ejection fraction (HFrEF). In particular, Implantable Cardioverter-Defibrillators (ICD) and Cardiac Resynchronization Therapy (CRT) may improve ejection fraction by reestablishing mechanical synchrony, possibly reversing symptoms and signs of heart failure, in addition to the more obvious role of ICD in terminating ventricular arrhythmias that threaten sudden death. Recommendations on device therapy from the current guidelines on heart failure management put out by the ESC/HFA in 2016[5] update our understanding of the evidence base for the use of ICD and CRT in HFrEF.

ICD

ICD's are pacemaker-like devices, originally developed in the 1970s for the electrical termination of ventricular tachyarrhythmias.[6] This technology has undergone considerable advances in the procedure of implantation, size and function. Whereas ICD's initially required invasive procedures for implantation (i.e. thoracotomy), advances in microprocessor technology have made the devices progressively smaller and therefore more easily implantable in the pectoral region with a per-cutaneous procedure. This procedure often lasts about 1 hour under local anesthesia. The ICD is composed of a microprocessor, batteries, capacitors and a "header" that contains a site to attach leads.[7] Different types of ICDs exist: single-chamber (one lead is placed in the right ventricle), dual-chamber (one right atrial lead and one right ventricular lead), and CRT ICDs (with also a left ventricular lead that is placed via the coronary sinus or epicardially).

Modern ICD's or mixed function devices now frequently fulfill multiple life-saving or disease modifying functions including atrial and ventricular defibrillation, anti-tachycardia pacing, backup bradycardia pacing, electrogram storage, and biventricular pacing.[7] According to the new ESC guidelines,[5] ICD's may be used in selected patients with HFrEF with the following aims: for primary prevention of sudden cardiac death in symptomatic patients and for secondary prevention of sudden cardiac death in symptomatic patients. Recommendations from the ESC guidelines, combined with a consideration of the ESC/European Heart Rhythm Association guidelines on ventricular tachyarrhythmias and sudden cardiac death[8] are below described.

ICD treatment in asymptomatic low ejection fraction patients

Regardless of symptoms, ICD implantation is recommended to prolong survival in patients expected to live more than 12 months with left ventricular systolic dysfunction (LVEF ≤ 35%) of ischaemic or non-ischaemic origin, provided in the case of recent MI the patient is at least 40 days after the acute myocardial infarction. Studies have demonstrated that ICD reduces mortality rates in these patients.[11,12,4,9] Importantly it has been demonstrated that in the 40 days immediately post-MI ICD implantation does not improve prognosis[9,10] and therefore ICD therapy is not recommended during this 40-day window.

ICD treatment in symptomatic heart failure patients

For primary prevention, ESC guidelines recommend ICD in order to diminish the risk of sudden death and all-cause mortality in symptomatic patients with NYHA class II–III and LVEF ≤ 35% despite at least 3 months of optimal medical therapy, and if there is clinical evidence of the following criteria:

a) expectation of survival longer than 1 year with good functional status; b) ischaemic heart disease (unless patient has had a myocardial infarction in the prior 40 days, as above described); c) dilated cardiomyopathy. In fact, it has been found that ICD decreases the rate of sudden death for arrhythmia in patients with HFrEF.[13,14] Notably, mortality rates are associated with the severity of heart failure,[15] i.e. patients with worse heart failure obtain a greater benefit from ICD, in terms of survival. Similarly, patients with ischaemic heart disease receive a greater benefit from ICD as they are at greater risk of sudden death than patients with dilated cardiomyopathy.[14] However, ICD is not recommended in heart failure patients with an extremely short prognosis, ie NYHA class IV and severe symptoms that are pharmacologically resistant and are not candidates for CRT, a ventricular assist device, or cardiac transplantation. In these patients, ICD has been found not to be beneficial.[16–18]

ICDs may be also used for secondary prevention. The new guidelines state that ICD is recommended "to reduce the risk of sudden death and all-cause mortality in patients who have recovered from a ventricular arrhythmia causing haemodynamic instability, and who are expected to survive for > 1 year with good functional status".[5] In this case, an ICD should be considered with the aim of prolonging survival. Notably, studies have shown that survival benefit is less clear when LVEF is over 35% and that the presence of comorbidities affects survival within the following year.[19–20] Thus, it is pivotal to carefully assess these parameters and patient's quality of life before taking the clinical decision for an ICD.[5] Before replacing the generator, the patient must be re-assessed to monitor the clinical status, his/her needs and possible changes in treatment aims, in order to decide if continue or not ICD therapy.[21–23] Finally, a wearable ICD may be considered for a short period of time or as a bridge to cardiac transplantation in patients at risk of sudden cardiac death.[24]

CRT

CRT is a device that may be used to restore synchronization, i.e. the normally coordinated pumping action of the ventricles. Unlike other pacemakers, CRT has a third lead that is positioned in a vein on the outer surface of the left ventricle. Advances in CRT design and implantation have made the device smaller and more practical (e.g. battery life is longer).[25] Specifically, CRT sends small, undetectable electrical impulses to both lower chambers of the heart to help them beat together, simultaneously stimulating the left and right ventricles.[3] A coordinated pattern may be therefore reestablished, improving the heart's ability to pump blood and oxygen to the body.

The current ESC/HFA guidelines recommend CRT in selected HFrEF patients to improve symptomatology and reduce morbidity and mortality (see Figure 9.1).[5] CRT is recommended to reduce mortality and morbidity in symptomatic patients in sinus rhythm with QRS duration ≥ 150 msec, a LBBB pattern and LVEF ≤ 35% despite optimal medical therapy. The guidelines also indicate that the use of CRT should be considered for patients with the aforementioned characteristics and non-LBBB QRS morphology, despite slightly less evidence in such patients. CRT is also recommended in symptomatic patients with heart failure in sinus rhythm and with a QRS duration of 130–149 msec and a LBBB QRS morphology with LVEF ≤ 35% despite optimal medical therapy in order to improve symptoms and reduce morbidity and mortality. The use of CRT may also be considered for patients with these characteristics and a non-LBBB QRS morphology, but some inconsistencies in available data do not allow us to draw firm conclusions in such patients.[5]

In order to improve symptoms and reduce morbidity and mortality, CRT should be considered for patients with LVEF ≤ 35% in NYHA class III–IV despite optimal medical therapy, if the following conditions are satisfied: a) atrial fibrillation; b) QRS duration ≥130 msec; c) patient expected to return to sinus rhythm (or a bi-ventricular capture strategy has been set). Regardless of NYHA class, CRT (rather than right ventricular pacing) is recommended for patients with HFrEF who are candidates for ventricular pacing for high degree atrio-ventricular block in order to reduce morbidity. This also includes patients with atrial fibrillation.

Although there are some inconsistencies in the available studies, CRT may be considered for patients with HFrEF who have received a conventional pacemaker or an ICD and subsequently develop worsening heart failure (but not if they have stable heart failure) despite optimal medical therapy and if they present a high proportion of right ventricular pacing. Thus, CRT therapy may reduce all-cause mortality, including sudden cardiac death. It may also

Recommendations	Class[a]	Level[b]
CRT is recommended for symptomatic patients with HF in sinus rhythm with a QRS duration ≥150 msec and LBBB QRS morphology and with LVEF ≤35% despite OMT in order to improve symptoms and reduce morbidity and mortality.	I	A
CRT should be considered for symptomatic patients with HF in sinus rhythm with a QRS duration ≥150 msec and non-LBBB QRS morphology and with LVEF ≤35% despite OMT in order to improve symptoms and reduce morbidity and mortality.	IIa	B
CRT is recommended for symptomatic patients with HF in sinus rhythm with a QRS duration of 130–149 msec and LBBB QRS morphology and with LVEF ≤35% despite OMT in order to improve symptoms and reduce morbidity and mortality.	I	B
CRT may be considered for symptomatic patients with HF in sinus rhythm with a QRS duration of 130–149 msec and non-LBBB QRS morphology and with LVEF ≤35% despite OMT in order to improve symptoms and reduce morbidity and mortality.	IIb	B
CRT rather than RV pacing is recommended for patients with HFrEF regardless of NYHA class who have an indication for ventricular pacing and high degree AV block in order to reduce morbidity. This includes patients with AF (see Section 10.1).	I	A
CRT should be considered for patients with LVEF ≤35% in NYHA Class III–IV[d] despite OMT in order to improve symptoms and reduce morbidity and mortality, if they are in AF and have a QRS duration ≥130 msec provided a strategy to ensure bi-ventricular capture is in place or the patient is expected to return to sinus rhythm.	IIa	B
Patients with HFrEF who have received a conventional pacemaker or an ICD and subsequently develop worsening HF despite OMT and who have a high proportion of RV pacing may be considered for upgrade to CRT. This does not apply to patients with stable HF.	IIb	B
CRT is contra-indicated in patients with a QRS duration < 130 msec.	III	A

FIGURE 9.1 Tabular guidance for the use of CRT in HFrEF.[5]

improve hospitalisations in HFrEF patients.[25] However, a marked heterogeneity of response has been noted in clinical trials on CRT.[7,26]

Response to treatment and complications

The response to CRT implantation in heart failure varies considerably according to features such as sex, QRS and LBBB characteristics and the aetiology of the heart failure. Specifically, studies on CRT have found that men are less likely to respond than women, possibly due to a larger body and heart size.[27,28] QRS width and morphology appear to be related to a beneficial response to CRT. In particular, QRS duration has been consistently found to predict the effects of CRT on morbidity and mortality in patients with symptomatic HFrEF who are in sinus rhythm.[29] Whether LBBB morphology per predicts a more favourable response to CRT independent of QRS width is less clear.

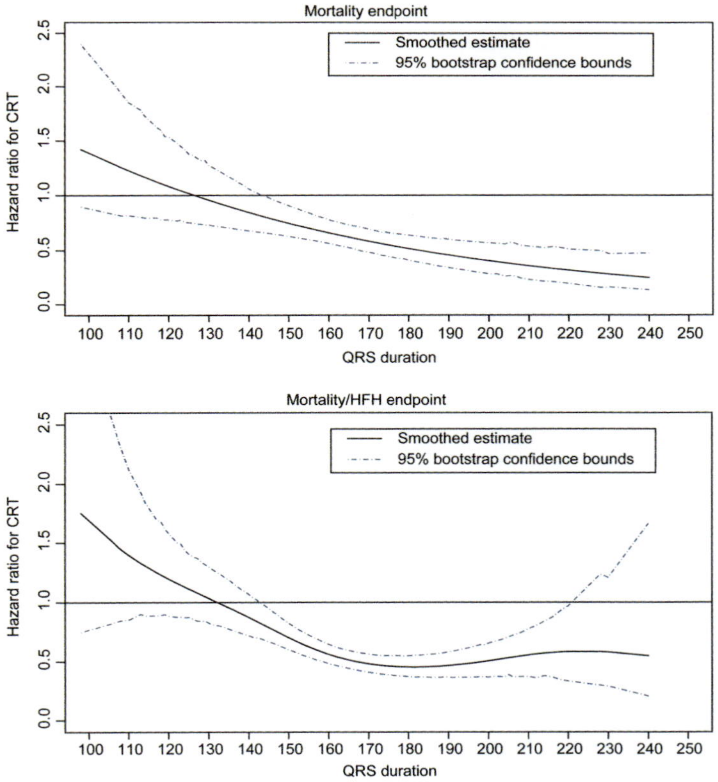

FIGURE 9.2 The impact of QRS duration on the reponse to CRT in HFpEF.[29]

The importance of QRS duration is evident from the individual patient meta-analysis performed by Cleland and colleagues (see Figure 9.2).

Patients with an ischaemic aetiology are less responsive, as the myocardial scar tissue is less amenable to effective remodelling.[30] These clinical features should be carefully assessed to understand clinical benefit versus implantation risks. In fact, a number of complications related to implantation and device activation have been described with the use of both devices.[7,31] Major complications include inappropriate shocks, device infection, lead malfunction and complications related to extraction of devices.[25] A harmful effect related to CRT has been found in patients with a QRS duration < 130 msec.[29,32,33] Thus, risk-benefit ratio of device therapy should be considered during clinical assessment and monitoring. Diminishing the implantation risks is a main challenge for upcoming research.

In conclusion, there is consistent evidence supporting the use of ICD and CRT in selected patients with HFrEF, to prolong life and avoid sudden death. With a strict application of the aforementioned recommendations from current guidelines, ICD and CRT treatments form an essential component of the modern management of patients with HFrEF.

References

1. Ukkonen, H., R. S. Beanlands, I. G. Burwash, R. A. de Kemp, C. Nahmias, E. Fallen, M. R. Hill and A. S. Tang (2003). Effect of cardiac resynchronization on myocardial efficiency and regional oxidative metabolism. Circulation 107(1): 28–31.
2. Biton, Y., J. R. Baman and B. Polonsky (2016). Roles and indications for use of implantable defibrillator and resynchronization therapy in the prevention of sudden cardiac death in heart failure. Heart Fail Rev.
3. Shea, J. B. and M. O. Sweeney (2003). Cardiology patient page. Cardiac resynchronization therapy: a patient's guide. Circulation 108(9): e64–66.
4. Kadish, A., A. Dyer, J. P. Daubert, R. Quigg, N. A. Estes, K. P. Anderson, H. Calkins, D. Hoch, J. Goldberger, A. Shalaby, W. E. Sanders, A. Schaechter, J. H. Levine and I. Defibrillators in Non-Ischemic Cardiomyopathy Treatment Evaluation (2004). Prophylactic defibrillator implantation in patients with nonischemic dilated cardiomyopathy. N Engl J Med 350(21): 2151–2158.
5. Ponikowski P, Voors AA, Anker SD, Bueno H, Cleland JG, Coats AJ, Falk V, González-Juanatey JR, Harjola VP, Jankowska EA, Jessup M, Linde C, Nihoyannopoulos P, Parissis JT, Pieske B, Riley JP, Rosano GM, Ruilope LM, Ruschitzka F, Rutten FH, van der Meer P; Authors/Task Force Members; Document Reviewers. 2016 ESC Guidelines for the diagnosis and treatment of acute and chronic heart failure: The Task Force for the diagnosis and treatment of acute and chronic heart failure of the European Society of Cardiology (ESC) Developed with the special contribution of the

Heart Failure Association (HFA) of the ESC. Eur Heart J. 2016 May 20. pii: ehw128. PMID: 27206819.

6. Mirowski, M. and M. M. Mower (1973). Transvenous automatic defibrillator as an approach to prevention of sudden death from ventricular fibrillation. Heart Lung 2(6): 867–869.
7. Kadish, A. and M. Mehra (2005). Heart failure devices: implantable cardioverter-defibrillators and biventricular pacing therapy. Circulation 111(24): 3327–3335.
8. Priori, S. G., C. Blomstrom-Lundqvist, A. Mazzanti, N. Blom, M. Borggrefe, J. Camm, P. M. Elliott, D. Fitzsimons, R. Hatala, G. Hindricks, P. Kirchhof, K. Kjeldsen, K. H. Kuck, A. Hernandez-Madrid, N. Nikolaou, T. M. Norekval, C. Spaulding and D. J. Van Veldhuisen (2015). 2015 ESC Guidelines for the management of patients with ventricular arrhythmias and the prevention of sudden cardiac death: The Task Force for the Management of Patients with Ventricular Arrhythmias and the Prevention of Sudden Cardiac Death of the European Society of Cardiology (ESC). Endorsed by: Association for European Paediatric and Congenital Cardiology (AEPC). Eur Heart J 36(41): 2793–2867.
9. Hohnloser, S. H., K. H. Kuck, P. Dorian, R. S. Roberts, J. R. Hampton, R. Hatala, E. Fain, M. Gent, S. J. Connolly and D. Investigators (2004). Prophylactic use of an implantable cardioverter-defibrillator after acute myocardial infarction. N Engl J Med 351(24): 2481–2488.
10. Steinbeck, G., D. Andresen, K. Seidl, J. Brachmann, E. Hoffmann, D. Wojciechowski, Z. Kornacewicz-Jach, B. Sredniawa, G. Lupkovics, F. Hofgartner, A. Lubinski, M. Rosenqvist, A. Habets, K. Wegscheider, J. Senges and I. Investigators (2009). Defibrillator implantation early after myocardial infarction. N Engl J Med 361(15): 1427–1436.
11. Moss, A. J., W. Zareba, W. J. Hall, H. Klein, D. J. Wilber, D. S. Cannom, J. P. Daubert, S. L. Higgins, M. W. Brown, M. L. Andrews and I. I. I. Multicenter Automatic Defibrillator Implantation Trial (2002). Prophylactic implantation of a defibrillator in patients with myocardial infarction and reduced ejection fraction. N Engl J Med 346(12): 877–883.
12. Desai, A. S., J. C. Fang, W. H. Maisel and K. L. Baughman (2004). Implantable defibrillators for the prevention of mortality in patients with nonischemic cardiomyopathy: a meta-analysis of randomized controlled trials. JAMA 292(23): 2874–2879.
13. Cook, N. R. and P. M. Ridker (2009). Advances in measuring the effect of individual predictors of cardiovascular risk: the role of reclassification measures. Ann Intern Med 150(11): 795–802.
14. Theuns, D. A., T. Smith, M. G. Hunink, G. H. Bardy and L. Jordaens (2010). Effectiveness of prophylactic implantation of cardioverter-defibrillators without cardiac resynchronization therapy in patients with ischaemic or non-ischaemic heart disease: a systematic review and meta-analysis. Europace 12(11): 1564–1570.
15. Bardy, G. H., K. L. Lee, D. B. Mark, J. E. Poole, D. L. Packer, R. Boineau, M. Domanski, C. Troutman, J. Anderson, G. Johnson, S. E. McNulty, N. Clapp-Channing, L. D. Davidson-Ray, E. S. Fraulo, D. P. Fishbein, R. M. Luceri, J. H. Ip and I.

Sudden Cardiac Death in Heart Failure Trial (2005). Amiodarone or an implantable cardioverter-defibrillator for congestive heart failure. N Engl J Med 352(3): 225–237.
16. Sanders, G. D., M. A. Hlatky and D. K. Owens (2005). Cost-effectiveness of implantable cardioverter-defibrillators. N Engl J Med 353(14): 1471–1480.
17. Miller, R. J., J. G. Howlett, D. V. Exner, P. M. Campbell, A. D. Grant and S. B. Wilton (2015). Baseline Functional Class and Therapeutic Efficacy of Common Heart Failure Interventions: A Systematic Review and Meta-analysis. Can J Cardiol 31(6): 792–799.
18. Raphael, C. E., J. A. Finegold, A. J. Barron, Z. I. Whinnett, J. Mayet, C. Linde, J. G. Cleland, W. C. Levy and D. P. Francis (2015). The effect of duration of follow-up and presence of competing risk on lifespan-gain from implantable cardioverter defibrillator therapy: who benefits the most? Eur Heart J 36(26): 1676–1688.
19. Connolly, S. J., M. Gent, R. S. Roberts, P. Dorian, D. Roy, R. S. Sheldon, L. B. Mitchell, M. S. Green, G. J. Klein and B. O'Brien (2000). Canadian implantable defibrillator study (CIDS) : a randomized trial of the implantable cardioverter defibrillator against amiodarone. Circulation 101(11): 1297–1302.
20. Connolly, S. J., A. P. Hallstrom, R. Cappato, E. B. Schron, K. H. Kuck, D. P. Zipes, H. L. Greene, S. Boczor, M. Domanski, D. Follmann, M. Gent and R. S. Roberts (2000). Meta-analysis of the implantable cardioverter defibrillator secondary prevention trials. AVID, CASH and CIDS studies. Antiarrhythmics vs Implantable Defibrillator study. Cardiac Arrest Study Hamburg. Canadian Implantable Defibrillator Study. Eur Heart J 21(24): 2071–2078.
21. Erkapic, D., J. Sperzel, S. Stiller, U. Meltendorf, J. Mermi, K. Wegscheider, B. Hugl and I. Investigators (2013). Long-term benefit of implantable cardioverter/defibrillator therapy after elective device replacement: results of the INcidence free SUrvival after ICD REplacement (INSURE) trial – a prospective multicentre study. Eur Heart J 34(2): 130–137.
22. Kini, V., M. K. Soufi, R. Deo, A. E. Epstein, R. Bala, M. Riley, P. W. Groeneveld, A. Shalaby and S. Dixit (2014). Appropriateness of primary prevention implantable cardioverter-defibrillators at the time of generator replacement: are indications still met? J Am Coll Cardiol 63(22): 2388–2394.
23. Yap, S. C., B. A. Schaer, R. E. Bhagwandien, M. Kuhne, L. Dabiri Abkenari, S. Osswald, T. Szili-Torok, C. Sticherling and D. A. Theuns (2014). Evaluation of the need of elective implantable cardioverter-defibrillator generator replacement in primary prevention patients without prior appropriate ICD therapy. Heart 100(15): 1188–1192.
24. Opreanu, M., C. Wan, V. Singh, N. Salehi, J. Ahmad, S. J. Szymkiewicz and R. K. Thakur (2015). Wearable cardioverter-defibrillator as a bridge to cardiac transplantation: A national database analysis. J Heart Lung Transplant 34(10): 1305–1309.
25. Kumar, P. and J. D. Schwartz (2015). Device therapies: new indications and future directions. Curr Cardiol Rev 11(1): 33–41.
26. Sohaib, S. M., J. A. Finegold, S. S. Nijjer, R. Hossain, C. Linde, W. C. Levy, R. Sutton, P. Kanagaratnam, D. P. Francis and Z. I. Whinnett (2015). Opportunity to increase life span in narrow QRS cardiac resynchronization therapy recipients by deactivating ventricular pacing: evidence from randomized controlled trials. JACC Heart Fail 3(4): 327–336.

27. Linde, C., M. Stahlberg, L. Benson, F. Braunschweig, M. Edner, U. Dahlstrom, U. Alehagen and L. H. Lund (2015). Gender, underutilization of cardiac resynchronization therapy, and prognostic impact of QRS prolongation and left bundle branch block in heart failure. Europace 17(3): 424–431.
28. Woods, B., N. Hawkins, S. Mealing, A. Sutton, W. T. Abraham, J. F. Beshai, H. Klein, M. Sculpher, C. J. Plummer and M. R. Cowie (2015). Individual patient data network meta-analysis of mortality effects of implantable cardiac devices. Heart 101(22): 1800–1806.
29. Cleland, J. G., W. T. Abraham, C. Linde, M. R. Gold, J. B. Young, J. Claude Daubert, L. Sherfesee, G. A. Wells and A. S. Tang (2013). An individual patient meta-analysis of five randomized trials assessing the effects of cardiac resynchronization therapy on morbidity and mortality in patients with symptomatic heart failure. Eur Heart J 34(46): 3547–3556.
30. Cleland, J. G., Y. Mareev and C. Linde (2015). Reflections on EchoCRT: sound guidance on QRS duration and morphology for CRT? Eur Heart J 36(30): 1948–1951.
31. Stewart, G. C., J. R. Weintraub, P. P. Pratibhu, M. J. Semigran, J. M. Camuso, K. Brooks, S. W. Tsang, M. S. Anello, V. T. Nguyen, E. F. Lewis, A. Nohria, A. S. Desai, M. M. Givertz and L. W. Stevenson (2010). Patient expectations from implantable defibrillators to prevent death in heart failure. J Card Fail 16(2): 106–113.
32. Ruschitzka, F., W. T. Abraham, J. P. Singh, J. J. Bax, J. S. Borer, J. Brugada, K. Dickstein, I. Ford, J. Gorcsan, 3rd, D. Gras, H. Krum, P. Sogaard, J. Holzmeister and C. R. T. S. G. Echo (2013). Cardiac-resynchronization therapy in heart failure with a narrow QRS complex. N Engl J Med 369(15): 1395–1405.
33. Steffel, J., M. Robertson, J. P. Singh, W. T. Abraham, J. J. Bax, J. S. Borer, K. Dickstein, I. Ford, J. Gorcsan, 3rd, D. Gras, H. Krum, P. Sogaard, J. Holzmeister, J. Brugada and F. Ruschitzka (2015). The effect of QRS duration on cardiac resynchronization therapy in patients with a narrow QRS complex: a subgroup analysis of the EchoCRT trial. Eur Heart J 36(30): 1983–1989.

10

Management of arrhythmias in heart failure

Introduction

Patients with heart failure (HF) often develop ventricular and supraventricular arrhythmias,[1] due in large part to electrical conduction abnormalities of the heart in this syndrome.[2] Cardiac remodeling and neurohumoral activation typical of HF create a substrate that increases the risk of developing arrhythmias and/or worsening pre-existing arrhythmias.[3] Advances in our understanding of the underlying pathophysiological mechanisms of HF have reinforced the importance of neurohumoral, mechanical and inflammatory processes as progressively more severe pump dysfunction occurs.[4] This combination increases the likelihood of arrhythmias, both atrial and ventricular, such that ventricular arrhythmias are found in up to 80% of patients with severe HF,[5] conferring additional risk of mortality and morbidity,[3] in particular via an increased risk of sudden cardiac death.[6–8] Arrhythmias are also responsible for an increased risk of rehospitalisation in one-third of HF patients.[9]

Arrhythmias include tachyarrhythmias (i.e. atrial, ventricular arrhythmias) and bradyarrhythmias (i.e. sinus node dysfunction, conduction disorders). Common HF-related supraventricular tachyarrhythmias include atrial fibrillation, atrial flutter, and paroxysmal supraventricular tachycardia. Ventricular arrhythmias include ventricular fibrillation and ventricular tachycardia.

The initial management of arrhythmias in HF requires identification and an accurate diagnosis. In this phase, ambulatory electrocardiographic examination may be required to detect and manage silent atrial fibrillation and monitor patients with suspected arrhythmia-related symptoms. Subsequent risk stratification can facilitate the assessment of the risk of sudden cardiac death or arterial embolism. Bleeding risk scores such as CHA2DS2-VASc and HAS-BLED scores should be administered as recommended in the ESC guidelines for atrial fibrillation (in press). Subsequently, a rate control strategy should be set, with a rhythm control strategy being reserved for patients with persistent arrhythmia-specific symptoms or if haemodynamically compromised by the arrhythmia (see below).

Atrial fibrillation in HF

The most common arrhythmia is atrial fibrillation, which is characterised by uncoordinated atrial activation with resultant impairment of atrial mechanical function.[10] Atrial fibrillation may be associated with other arrhythmias, most commonly atrial tachycardia or atrial flutter. Atrial tachycardia is a supraventricular tachycardia that originates from a "focus" or spot in the left or right atrium with a heart rate of > 100 beats per minute. Atrial flutter is characterised by atrial rates of 240–400 beats/min and some degree of atrio-ventricular node conduction block, with "flutter" waves on the ECG (i.e. a saw-tooth pattern of regular atrial activation). Atrial flutter may develop into atrial fibrillation and atrial fibrillation may reverse to atrial flutter.[10]

The prevalence of atrial fibrillation in HF outpatients ranges from 19 to 37%[10,11] but rises up to 50% in those recently hospitalised.[12,13] The prevalence of atrial fibrillation also increases with the severity of HF, with rates ranging from less than 5% in patients with NYHA Class I[14] to nearly 50% in Class IV.[15] Other associated characteristics are female gender, older age, a lower prevalence of coronary artery disease and higher prevalence of valvular heart disease or chronic non-cardiac diseases than HF patients without atrial fibrillation.[3]

HF is a recognised risk factor for atrial fibrillation[16] and the occurrence of atrial fibrillation is associated with increased mortality in HF.[17] A recent meta-analysis has shown that all-cause mortality due to incident atrial fibrillation is significantly higher in HF patients with reduced ejection fraction (HFrEF) compared to those with preserved ejection fraction (HFpEF).[18] Finally, even in the absence of overt clinical symptoms, atrial fibrillation predicts stroke and worsening of HF symptoms.[19,3]

Nearly 40% of patients with atrial fibrillation go on to develop HF.[13] and the incident HF is associated with worse symptomatology[20] and increased mortality.[17] However, atrial fibrillation in isolation has not been consistently found to be a risk factor for HF independent of other possibly shared risk factors.[21–24] Thus, HF and atrial fibrillation often co-exist, and this may be explained considering common risk factors and intertwining, self-perpetuating processes.[3]

In the clinical management of HF it is important, although challenging, to identify whether HF is a trigger or a consequence of atrial fibrillation.

Management of atrial fibrillation in HF

Atrial fibrillation may be treated with drugs to slow the heart rate ("rate control") or to convert the rhythm to normal sinus rhythm ("rhythm control"). Electrical cardioversion may be used for rhythm control especially when the clinical status is not stable.[10] Ablation may be a strategy for relapse prevention in patients with HF and HFrEF, chronic atrial fibrillation and controlled ventricular rate.[3]

In patients with HFpEF and atrial fibrillation there is a more complicated phenotype[25] characterised by increased pulmonary artery pressure, higher biomarker levels and worse systolic function than HFpEF patients without atrial fibrillation.[19] Due to this worse clinical status, HFpEF patients with atrial fibrillation are at higher risk of mortality and hospitalisation than those without atrial fibrillation.[26,27]

Updated evidence-based recommendations for the management of atrial fibrillation in HF have been developed by the 2016 ESC guidelines on HF.[28] The recent ESC/HFA recommendations for the management of atrial fibrillation in HF are reproduced in Figure 10.1. Notably, ACEI, ARB, beta-blockers and MRA may be used to prevent atrial fibrillation in HF, but ivabradine is not indicated as it may increase its incidence.[29] Rate control should be documented by ECG and the preferred ventricular rate at rest is 60–100 bpm according to the ESC/HFA guidelines,[28] although more studies are probably needed for accurate targeting of preferred AF rates. Despite the fact that the optimal strategy to control ventricular rate remains elusive, beta-blockers, digoxin and the combination may be used[30] with beta-blockers the preferred first-line agent.[28] A rhythm control strategy (including pharmacological or electrical cardioversion) has not been shown to be superior to a rate control strategy in reducing mortality or morbidity in chronic HF,[31] and is indicated only if atrial fibrillation is life threatening or specifically related to disabling symptoms.[28]

Ventricular arrhythmias in HF

Ventricular arrhythmias include several different clinical pictures, spanning from isolated and asymptomatic ventricular ectopy at ECG to fatal ventricular fibrillation. Ventricular arrhythmias are common in chronic HF, particularly in patients with HFrEF. The risk of ventricular arrhythmias is higher in HF patients with an ischaemic aetiology[32] and in those with concurrent comorbidities.[3] According to the 2016 ESC/HFA guidelines, the management

Recommendations	Class[a]	Level[b]
Urgent electrical cardioversion is recommended if AF is thought to be contributing to the patient's haemodynamic compromise in order to improve the patient clinical condition.	I	C
For patients in NYHA Class IV, in addition to treatment for AHF, an intravenous bolus of amiodarone or, in digoxin-naïve patients, an intravenous bolus of digoxin should be considered to reduce the ventricular rate.	IIa	B
For patients in NYHA Class I–III, a beta-blocker, usually given orally, is safe and therefore is recommended as first-line treatment to control ventricular rate, provided the patient is euvolaemic.	I	A
For patients in NYHA Class I–III, digoxin, should be considered when ventricular rate remains high[d] despite beta-blockers or when beta-blockers are not tolerated or contra-indicated.	IIa	B
AV node catheter ablation may be considered to control heart rate and relieve symptoms in patients unresponsive or intolerant to intensive pharmacological rate and rhythm control therapy, accepting that these patients will become pacemaker dependent.	IIb	B
Treatment with dronedarone to improve ventricular rate control is not recommended due to safety concerns.	III	A

FIGURE 10.1A Recommendations for initial management of a rapid ventricular rate in patients with heart failure & atrial fibrillation in the acute or chronic setting.[28]

AF = atrial fibrillation; AHF= acute heart failure; AV= atrio-ventricular; bpm = beats per minute

Recommendations	Class [a]	Level [b]
Electrical cardioversion or pharmacological cardioversion with amiodarone may be considered in patients with persisting symptoms and/or signs of HF, despite OMT and adequate control of ventricular rate, to improve clinical/symptomatic status.	IIb	B
AF ablation may be considered in order to restore sinus rhythm to improve symptoms in patients with persisting symptoms and/or signs of HF, despite OMT and adequate control of ventricular rate, to improve clinical/symptomatic status.	IIb	B
Amiodarone may be considered prior to (and following) successful electrical cardioversion to maintain sinus rhythm.	IIb	B
Dronedarone is not recommended because of an increased risk of hospital admissions for cardiovascular causes and an increased risk of premature death in NYHA Class III–IV patients.	III	A
Class I antiarrhythmic agents are not recommended because of an increased risk of premature death.	III	A

FIGURE 10.1B Recommendations for a rhythm control management strategy in patients with atrial fibrillation, symptomatic heart failure (NYHA Class II–IV) & left ventricular systolic dysfunction and no evidence of acute decompensation.[28]

* The optimal ventricular rate for patients with HF and AF has not been established but the range of 60–100 bpm is currently recommended by the ESC guidelines.

Recommendations	Class[a]	Level[b]
The CHA_2DS_2-VASc and HAS-BLED scores are recommended tools in patients with HF for the estimation of the risk of thromboembolism and the risk of bleeding associated with oral anticoagulation, respectively.	I	B
An oral anticoagulant is recommended to prevent thrombo-embolism for all patients with paroxysmal or persistent/permanent AF and a CHA_2DS_2-VASc score ≥2, without contra-indications, and irrespective of whether a rate or rhythm management strategy is used (including after successful cardioversion).	I	A
NOAC treatment is contra-indicated in patients with mechanical valves or at least moderate mitral stenosis.	III	B
In patients with AF of ≥48 h duration, or when the duration of AF is unknown, an oral anticoagulant is recommended at a therapeutic dose for ≥3 weeks prior to electrical or pharmacological cardioversion.	I	B
Intravenous heparin or LMWH and TOE quided strategy is recommended for patients who have not been treated with an anticoagulant dose for ≥3 weeks and require urgent electrical or pharmacological cardioversion for a life threatening arrhythmia.	I	C
Combination of an oral anticoagulant and an antiplatelet agent is not recommended in patients with chronic (>12 months after an acute event) coronary or other arterial disease, because of a high-risk of serious bleeding. Single therapy with an oral anticoagulant is preferred after 12 months.	III	C
For patients with HF and non-valvular AF eligible for anticoagulation based on a CHA_2DS_2-VASc score, NOACs rather than warfarin should be considered for anticoagulation as NOACs are associated with a lower risk of stroke, intracranial haemorrhage and mortality, which outweigh the increased risk of gastrointestinal haemorrhage.	IIa	B

FIGURE 10.1C Recommendations for the prevention of thromboembolism in patients with symptomatic HF (NYHA Class II–IV) and paroxysmal or persistent/permanent AF.[28]

CHA_2DS_2-VASc = Congestive heart failure or left ventricular dysfunction, Hypertension, Age ≥ 75 (doubled), Diabetes, Stroke (doubled)-Vascular disease, Age 65–74, Sex category (female); HAS-BLED = Hypertension, Abnormal renal/liver function (1 point each), Stroke, Bleeding history or predisposition, Labile international normalised ratio, Elderly (> 65 years), Drugs/alcohol concomitantly (1 point each); HF = heart failure; LMWH = low molecular weight heparin; LVSD= left ventricular systolic dysfunction; NOAC = non-vitamin K antagonist oral anticoagulant; NYHA = New York Heart Association; OMT= optimal medical therapy; TOE = transoesophageal echocardiography.

of asymptomatic ventricular arrhythmias starts with correction of precipitants such as electrolyte abnormalities (low serum potassium and magnesium), interruption of potentially arrhythmogenic agents and optimisation of pharmacological therapy. In particular, since ventricular arrhythmias are associated with an increased risk of sudden death, ACEIs, beta-blockers, MRA and LCZ696 may be used for prevention in patients with HFrEF.[28] Other antiarrhythmic drugs (e.g. amiodarone in the setting severe HF) should be avoided as they may affect adversely the prognosis.[6,33–34] Implantable cardioverter defibrillators should also be used to reduce the risk of sudden death in selected patients (see Chapter 9). Updated evidence-based recommendations for the management of ventricular tachyarrhythmias in HF developed by the 2016 ESC guidelines are listed in Table 10.1.

Symptomatic bradycardia, pauses and atrio-ventricular block in HF

Patients with HF are often characterised by bradyarrhythmias and pauses, occurring in particular during the night (due to the drop of sympathetic

TABLE 10.1 Recommendations for the management of ventricular tachyarrhythmias in HF from the ESC/HFA guidelines[28]

Recommendation	Class
Potential aggravating/precipitating factors (e.g. low serum potassium/magnesium, ongoing ischaemia) should be considered to be sought and corrected in patients with ventricular arrhythmias.	IIa
Treatment with an ACEI (or ARB), beta-blocker, and MRA in optimal doses reduces risk for SCD and is recommended for patients with HFrEF and ventricular arrhythmias (as for other patients).	I
Implantation of an ICD or CRT-D device is recommended for selected patients with HFrEF.	I
Several strategies should be considered to reduce recurrent symptomatic arrhythmias in patients with an ICD (or in those who are not eligible for ICD), including attention to risk factors and optimal pharmacological treatment of HF, amiodarone, catheter ablation and CRT.	IIa
Routine use of antiarrhythmic agents is not recommended in patients with HF and asymptomatic ventricular arrhythmias because of safety concerns (worsening HF, proarrhythmia, and death).	III

Class of recommendation: I= evidence and/or general agreement that a given treatment or procedure is beneficial, useful, effective; II= conflicting evidence and/or a divergence of opinion about the usefulness/efficacy of the given treatment or procedure (IIa: weight of evidence/opinion is in favor of usefulness/efficacy; IIb: usefulness/efficacy is less well established by evidence/opinion); III: evidence or general agreement that the given treatment or procedure is not useful/effective, and in some cases may be harmful.

ACEI = angiotensin-converting enzyme inhibitor; ARB = angiotensin receptor blocker; CRT = cardiac resynchronization therapy; CRT-D = defibrillator with cardiac resynchronization therapy; HF = heart failure; HFrEF = heart failure with reduced ejection fraction; ICD = implantable cardioverter defibrillator; MRA = mineralocorticoid receptor antagonist.

activity and the rise of parasympathetic activity), and may be triggered by sleep apnoea.[35–37] Pauses and bradycardia may lead to a worse prognosis in HF. In particular, intermittent high-degree atrioventricular block[38] and bradycardia[39] are associated with a high risk of cardiac death in HF patients. Pacing devices as recommended for prevention by current ESC/ European Heart Rhythm Association (EHRA) guidelines on cardiac pacing and cardiac resynchronization therapy.[40] ICDs with pacemaker function (see Chapter 9) have been demonstrated to be effective for the prevention of bradycardia, beyond the correction of ventricular arrhythmias. In particular, ESC/EHRA guidelines recommend intervention for pauses over 6 seconds in the absence of myocardial dysfunction. On the other hand, in patients with HFrEF also shorter pauses require intervention.[38] For the treatment of bradycardic pauses >3 seconds or symptomatic bradycardia of rate <50 bpm in sinus rhythm or <60 in AF the need for and dose of bardycardiac medication should be reviewed. In HF patients with symptomatic, prolonged or frequent pauses despite adjustment of rate limiting medication, the next steps to be considered include either beta-blocker withdrawal or back-up pacing, although pacing solely to permit initiation or up-titration of beta-blockers is not recommended. In HFrEF patients who do have a compelling indication for pacing in the presence of high degree AV block, CRT rather than RV pacing is recommended, and in the absence of high degree AV block, pacing modes that avoid inducing or exacerbating ventricular dyssynchrony should be considered.

Arrhythmias in acute HF

Acute HF may present with severe rhythm disturbances that should be corrected immediately by pharmacotherapy, electrical cardioversion and/or temporary pacing[28,40,41] especially if (whether atrial or ventricular) is thought to be contributing to the patient's haemodynamic distress. Rate control should be preferred in acute HF, followed by a rhythm control strategy after the acute phase of HF has resolved.[3] Some patients with acute HF may have persistent ventricular arrhythmias; the latter often perpetuates haemodynamic instability and *vice versa*. In this case, immediate angiography and electrophysiological testing with radiofrequency ablation may be considered.[41]

Conclusions

The high risk of arrhythmias should always be considered during the clinical management of all HF patients, due their association with worse prognosis and increased mortality. In particular, HF and atrial fibrillation mutually worsen the impact of each other. Treatment of atrial fibrillation in the setting of HF includes a variety of approaches such as drugs, devices and ablation. Restoration of sinus rhythm is not superior to optimal rate control, and the deleterious effects of antiarrhythmic drugs should be considered. Finally, cardiac function, symptoms, and quality of life may improve with catheter-based ablative therapies in appropriately selected patients with HF.[42]

References

1. Luong, C., M. E. Barnes and T. S. Tsang (2014). Atrial fibrillation and heart failure: cause or effect? Curr Heart Fail Rep 11(4): 463–470.
2. Dean, J. W. and M. J. Lab (1989). Arrhythmia in heart failure: role of mechanically induced changes in electrophysiology. Lancet 1(8650): 1309–1312.

3. Lip, G. Y., F. R. Heinzel, F. Gaita, J. R. Juanatey, J. Y. Le Heuzey, T. Potpara, J. H. Svendsen, M. A. Vos, S. D. Anker, A. J. Coats, W. Haverkamp, A. S. Manolis, M. K. Chung, P. Sanders and B. Pieske (2015). European Heart Rhythm Association/Heart Failure Association joint consensus document on arrhythmias in heart failure, endorsed by the Heart Rhythm Society and the Asia Pacific Heart Rhythm Society. Eur J Heart Fail 17(9): 848–874.
4. Fang, J. C., G. A. Ewald, L. A. Allen, J. Butler, C. A. Westlake Canary, M. Colvin-Adams, M. G. Dickinson, P. Levy, W. G. Stough, N. K. Sweitzer, J. R. Teerlink, D. J. Whellan, N. M. Albert, R. Krishnamani, M. W. Rich, M. N. Walsh, M. R. Bonnell, P. E. Carson, M. C. Chan, D. L. Dries, A. F. Hernandez, R. E. Hershberger, S. D. Katz, S. Moore, J. E. Rodgers, J. G. Rogers, A. R. Vest, M. M. Givertz and C. Heart Failure Society of America Guidelines (2015). Advanced (stage D) heart failure: a statement from the Heart Failure Society of America Guidelines Committee. J Card Fail 21(6): 519–534.
5. Singh, S. N., P. E. Carson and S. G. Fisher (1997). Nonsustained ventricular tachycardia in severe heart failure. Circulation 96(10): 3794–3795.
6. Bardy, G. H., K. L. Lee, D. B. Mark, J. E. Poole, D. L. Packer, R. Boineau, M. Domanski, C. Troutman, J. Anderson, G. Johnson, S. E. McNulty, N. Clapp-Channing, L. D. Davidson-Ray, E. S. Fraulo, D. P. Fishbein, R. M. Luceri, J. H. Ip and I. Sudden Cardiac Death in Heart Failure Trial (2005). Amiodarone or an implantable cardioverter-defibrillator for congestive heart failure. N Engl J Med 352(3): 225–237.
7. Lane, R. E., M. R. Cowie and A. W. Chow (2005). Prediction and prevention of sudden cardiac death in heart failure. Heart 91(5): 674–680.
8. Ramineni, R., M. K. Bheemarasetti, A. Baranchuk, T. Mandalapu, V. K. Mukku, K. Fujise and A. Barbagelata (2012). Management of arrhythmias in heart failure. What a practicing physician should know in the current times. Cardiol J 19(6): 567–577.
9. Nieminen, M. S., D. Brutsaert, K. Dickstein, H. Drexler, F. Follath, V. P. Harjola, M. Hochadel, M. Komajda, J. Lassus, J. L. Lopez-Sendon, P. Ponikowski, L. Tavazzi, I. EuroHeart Survey and E. S. o. C. Heart Failure Association (2006). EuroHeart Failure Survey II (EHFS II): a survey on hospitalized acute heart failure patients: description of population. Eur Heart J 27(22): 2725–2736.
10. Fuster, V., L. E. Ryden, D. S. Cannom, et al. ACC/AHA/ESC 2006 guidelines for the management of patients with atrial fibrillation: full text: a report of the American College of Cardiology/American Heart Association Task Force on practice guidelines and the European Society of Cardiology Committee for Practice Guidelines (Writing Committee to Revise the 2001 guidelines for the management of patients with atrial fibrillation) developed in collaboration with the European Heart Rhythm Association and the Heart Rhythm Society. Europace 8(9): 651–745.
11. Corell, P., F. Gustafsson, M. Schou, J. Markenvard, T. Nielsen and P. Hildebrandt (2007). Prevalence and prognostic significance of atrial fibrillation in outpatients with heart failure due to left ventricular systolic dysfunction. Eur J Heart Fail 9(3): 258–265.
12. Maggioni, A. P., U. Dahlstrom, G. Filippatos, O. Chioncel, M. Crespo Leiro, J. Drozdz, F. Fruhwald, L. Gullestad, D. Logeart, G. Fabbri, R. Urso, M. Metra, J. Parissis, H. Persson, P. Ponikowski, M. Rauchhaus, A. A. Voors, O. W. Nielsen, F. Zannad, L. Tavazzi and C. Heart Failure Association of the European Society of (2013). EURObservational

Research Programme: regional differences and 1-year follow-up results of the Heart Failure Pilot Survey (ESC-HF Pilot). Eur J Heart Fail 15(7): 808–817.
13. Ambrosy, A. P., G. C. Fonarow, J. Butler, O. Chioncel, S. J. Greene, M. Vaduganathan, S. Nodari, C. S. Lam, N. Sato, A. N. Shah and M. Gheorghiade (2014). The global health and economic burden of hospitalizations for heart failure: lessons learned from hospitalized heart failure registries. J Am Coll Cardiol 63(12): 1123–1133.
14. The SOLVD Investigators. (1992). Effect of enalapril on mortality and the development of heart failure in asymptomatic patients with reduced left ventricular ejection fractions. N Engl J Med 327(10): 685–691.
15. The CONSENSUS Trial Study Group. Effects of enalapril on mortality in severe congestive heart failure. Results of the Cooperative North Scandinavian Enalapril Survival Study (CONSENSUS). N Engl J Med 316(23): 1429–1435.
16. Schnabel, R. B., L. M. Sullivan, D. Levy, M. J. Pencina, J. M. Massaro, R. B. D'Agostino, Sr., C. Newton-Cheh, J. F. Yamamoto, J. W. Magnani, T. M. Tadros, W. B. Kannel, T. J. Wang, P. T. Ellinor, P. A. Wolf, R. S. Vasan and E. J. Benjamin (2009). Development of a risk score for atrial fibrillation (Framingham Heart Study): a community-based cohort study. Lancet 373(9665): 739–745.
17. Wang, T. J., M. G. Larson, D. Levy, R. S. Vasan, E. P. Leip, P. A. Wolf, R. B. D'Agostino, J. M. Murabito, W. B. Kannel and E. J. Benjamin (2003). Temporal relations of atrial fibrillation and congestive heart failure and their joint influence on mortality: the Framingham Heart Study. Circulation 107(23): 2920–2925.
18. Kotecha, D., R. Chudasama, D. A. Lane, P. Kirchhof and G. Y. Lip (2016). Atrial fibrillation and heart failure due to reduced versus preserved ejection fraction: A systematic review and meta-analysis of death and adverse outcomes. Int J Cardiol 203: 660–666.
19. Zakeri, R., B. A. Borlaug, S. E. McNulty, S. F. Mohammed, G. D. Lewis, M. J. Semigran, A. Deswal, M. LeWinter, A. F. Hernandez, E. Braunwald and M. M. Redfield (2014). Impact of atrial fibrillation on exercise capacity in heart failure with preserved ejection fraction: a RELAX trial ancillary study. Circ Heart Fail 7(1): 123–130.
20. Agostoni, P., M. Emdin, U. Corra, F. Veglia, D. Magri, C. C. Tedesco, E. Berton, C. Passino, E. Bertella, F. Re, A. Mezzani, R. Belardinelli, C. Colombo, R. La Gioia, M. Vicenzi, A. Giannoni, D. Scrutinio, P. Giannuzzi, C. Tondo, A. Di Lenarda, G. Sinagra, M. F. Piepoli and M. Guazzi (2008). Permanent atrial fibrillation affects exercise capacity in chronic heart failure patients. Eur Heart J 29(19): 2367–2372.
21. Rivero-Ayerza, M., W. Scholte Op Reimer, M. Lenzen, D. A. Theuns, L. Jordaens, M. Komajda, F. Follath, K. Swedberg and J. G. Cleland (2008). New-onset atrial fibrillation is an independent predictor of in-hospital mortality in hospitalized heart failure patients: results of the EuroHeart Failure Survey. Eur Heart J 29(13): 1618–1624.
22. Santini, M., M. Gasparini, M. Landolina, M. Lunati, A. Proclemer, L. Padeletti, D. Catanzariti, G. Molon, G. L. Botto, L. La Rocca, A. Grammatico, G. Boriani and P. cardiological centers participating in ClinicalService (2011). Device-detected atrial tachyarrhythmias predict adverse outcome in real-world patients with implantable biventricular defibrillators. J Am Coll Cardiol 57(2): 167–172.
23. Lam, C. S., P. E. Carson, I. S. Anand, T. S. Rector, M. Kuskowski, M. Komajda, R. S. McKelvie, J. J. McMurray, M. R. Zile, B. M. Massie and D. W. Kitzman (2012). Sex differences in clinical characteristics and outcomes in elderly patients with heart

failure and preserved ejection fraction: the Irbesartan in Heart Failure with Preserved Ejection Fraction (I-PRESERVE) trial. Circ Heart Fail 5(5): 571–578.

24. Mentz, R. J., M. J. Chung, M. Gheorghiade, P. S. Pang, M. J. Kwasny, A. P. Ambrosy, M. Vaduganathan, C. M. O'Connor, K. Swedberg, F. Zannad, M. A. Konstam and A. P. Maggioni (2012). Atrial fibrillation or flutter on initial electrocardiogram is associated with worse outcomes in patients admitted for worsening heart failure with reduced ejection fraction: findings from the EVEREST Trial. Am Heart J 164(6): 884–892 e882.
25. Nanayakkara, S. and D. M. Kaye (2015). Management of heart failure with preserved ejection fraction: a review. Clin Ther 37(10): 2186–2198.
26. Linssen, G. C., M. Rienstra, T. Jaarsma, A. A. Voors, I. C. van Gelder, H. L. Hillege and D. J. van Veldhuisen (2011). Clinical and prognostic effects of atrial fibrillation in heart failure patients with reduced and preserved left ventricular ejection fraction. Eur J Heart Fail 13(10): 1111–1120.
27. Taillandier, S., A. Brunet Bernard, B. Lallemand, E. Simeon, L. Pericart, N. Clementy, D. Babuty and L. Fauchier (2014). Prognosis in patients hospitalized with permanent and nonpermanent atrial fibrillation in heart failure. Am J Cardiol 113(7): 1189–1195.
28. Ponikowski P, Voors AA, Anker SD, Bueno H, Cleland JG, Coats AJ, Falk V, González-Juanatey JR, Harjola VP, Jankowska EA, Jessup M, Linde C, Nihoyannopoulos P, Parissis JT, Pieske B, Riley JP, Rosano GM, Ruilope LM, Ruschitzka F, Rutten FH, van der Meer P; Authors/Task Force Members; Document Reviewers. 2016 ESC Guidelines for the diagnosis and treatment of acute and chronic heart failure: The Task Force for the diagnosis and treatment of acute and chronic heart failure of the European Society of Cardiology (ESC) Developed with the special contribution of the Heart Failure Association (HFA) of the ESC. Eur Heart J. 2016 May 20. pii: ehw128. PMID: 27206819.
29. Martin, R. I., O. Pogoryelova, M. S. Koref, J. P. Bourke, M. D. Teare and B. D. Keavney (2014). Atrial fibrillation associated with ivabradine treatment: meta-analysis of randomised controlled trials. Heart 100(19): 1506–1510.
30. Khand, A. U., A. C. Rankin, W. Martin, J. Taylor, I. Gemmell and J. G. Cleland (2003). Carvedilol alone or in combination with digoxin for the management of atrial fibrillation in patients with heart failure? J Am Coll Cardiol 42(11): 1944–1951.
31. Roy, D., M. Talajic, S. Nattel, D. G. Wyse, P. Dorian, K. L. Lee, M. G. Bourassa, J. M. Arnold, A. E. Buxton, A. J. Camm, S. J. Connolly, M. Dubuc, A. Ducharme, P. G. Guerra, S. H. Hohnloser, J. Lambert, J. Y. Le Heuzey, G. O'Hara, O. D. Pedersen, J. L. Rouleau, B. N. Singh, L. W. Stevenson, W. G. Stevenson, B. Thibault, A. L. Waldo, F. Atrial and I. Congestive Heart Failure (2008). Rhythm control versus rate control for atrial fibrillation and heart failure. N Engl J Med 358(25): 2667–2677.
32. Gupta, S. and V. M. Figueredo (2014). Tachycardia mediated cardiomyopathy: pathophysiology, mechanisms, clinical features and management. Int J Cardiol 172(1): 40–46.
33. Torp-Pedersen, C., M. Metra, P. Spark, M. A. Lukas, C. Moullet, A. Scherhag, M. Komajda, J. G. Cleland, W. Remme, A. Di Lenarda, K. Swedberg, P. A. Poole-Wilson and C. Investigators (2007). The safety of amiodarone in patients with heart failure. J Card Fail 13(5): 340–345.
34. Kober, L., C. Torp-Pedersen, J. J. McMurray, O. Gotzsche, S. Levy, H. Crijns, J. Amlie,

J. Carlsen and G. Dronedarone Study (2008). Increased mortality after dronedarone therapy for severe heart failure. N Engl J Med 358(25): 2678–2687.

35. Cintra, F. D., R. P. Leite, L. J. Storti, L. A. Bittencourt, D. Poyares, L. D. Castro, S. Tufik and A. D. Paola (2014). Sleep Apnea and Nocturnal Cardiac Arrhythmia: A Populational Study. Arq Bras Cardiol 103(5): 368–374.
36. Gilat, H., S. Vinker, I. Buda, E. Soudry, M. Shani and G. Bachar (2014). Obstructive sleep apnea and cardiovascular comorbidities: a large epidemiologic study. Medicine (Baltimore) 93(9): e45.
37. Vizzardi, E., E. Sciatti, I. Bonadei, A. D'Aloia, A. Curnis and M. Metra (2014). Obstructive sleep apnoea-hypopnoea and arrhythmias: new updates. J Cardiovasc Med (Hagerstown).
38. Bloch Thomsen, P. E., C. Jons, M. J. Raatikainen, R. Moerch Joergensen, J. Hartikainen, V. Virtanen, J. Boland, O. Anttonen, U. J. Gang, N. Hoest, L. V. Boersma, E. S. Platou, D. Becker, M. D. Messier, H. V. Huikuri, A. Cardiac and G. Risk Stratification After Acute Myocardial Infarction Study (2010). Long-term recording of cardiac arrhythmias with an implantable cardiac monitor in patients with reduced ejection fraction after acute myocardial infarction: the Cardiac Arrhythmias and Risk Stratification After Acute Myocardial Infarction (CARISMA) study. Circulation 122(13): 1258–1264.
39. Faggiano, P., A. d'Aloia, A. Gualeni, A. Gardini and A. Giordano (2001). Mechanisms and immediate outcome of in-hospital cardiac arrest in patients with advanced heart failure secondary to ischemic or idiopathic dilated cardiomyopathy. Am J Cardiol 87(5): 655–657, A610–651.
40. Brignole, M., A. Auricchio, G. Baron-Esquivias, et al. (2013). 2013 ESC Guidelines on cardiac pacing and cardiac resynchronization therapy: the Task Force on cardiac pacing and resynchronization therapy of the European Society of Cardiology (ESC). Developed in collaboration with the European Heart Rhythm Association (EHRA). Eur Heart J 34(29): 2281–2329.
41. Priori, S. G., C. Blomstrom-Lundqvist, A. Mazzanti, N. Blom, M. Borggrefe, J. Camm, P. M. Elliott, D. Fitzsimons, R. Hatala, G. Hindricks, P. Kirchhof, K. Kjeldsen, K. H. Kuck, A. Hernandez-Madrid, N. Nikolaou, T. M. Norekval, C. Spaulding and D. J. Van Veldhuisen (2015). 2015 ESC Guidelines for the management of patients with ventricular arrhythmias and the prevention of sudden cardiac death: The Task Force for the Management of Patients with Ventricular Arrhythmias and the Prevention of Sudden Cardiac Death of the European Society of Cardiology (ESC). Endorsed by: Association for European Paediatric and Congenital Cardiology (AEPC). Eur Heart J 36(41): 2793–2867.
42. Anter, E., M. Jessup and D. J. Callans (2009). Atrial fibrillation and heart failure: treatment considerations for a dual epidemic. Circulation 119(18): 2516–2525.

11

Other devices – cardiac contractility modulation (CCM)

Introduction

Substantial advances in the medical treatment of HFrEF have improved survival and cardiac function in these patients. However despite the use of optimal medical therapy (OMT) and the use of recommended devices in those in whom they are indicated, persistent symptoms limit activity and adversely affect lifestyle in a substantial number of patients. For these patients newer devices other than ICD and CRT may offer an improvement in symptoms and/or survival. The recent 2016 ESC/HFA guidelines for the management of heart failure[1] considered that most of these newer devices had insufficient clinical trial data for a formal recommendation, but in the case of one, cardiac contractility modulation (CCM) the guidelines describe CCM as being something to be considered in selected patients with HF. This is based on a demonstrated improvement in exercise tolerance (peak VO_2) and quality of life (by Minnesota LWHF questionnaire, MLWHFQ) produced by CCM in an individual patient data meta-analysis of all the randomised controlled trials of CCM.[2] We review in this chapter the evidence for the use of CCM and discuss in which patients it may be considered as recommended in the recent guidelines.

Is there a need for novel devices?

Approximately half of heart failure patients receiving OMT with persistent and restrictive symptoms (NHYA II-IV) have EF<35% and are candidates for ICD (Figure 11.1). Of these, approximately one third have LBBB or wide

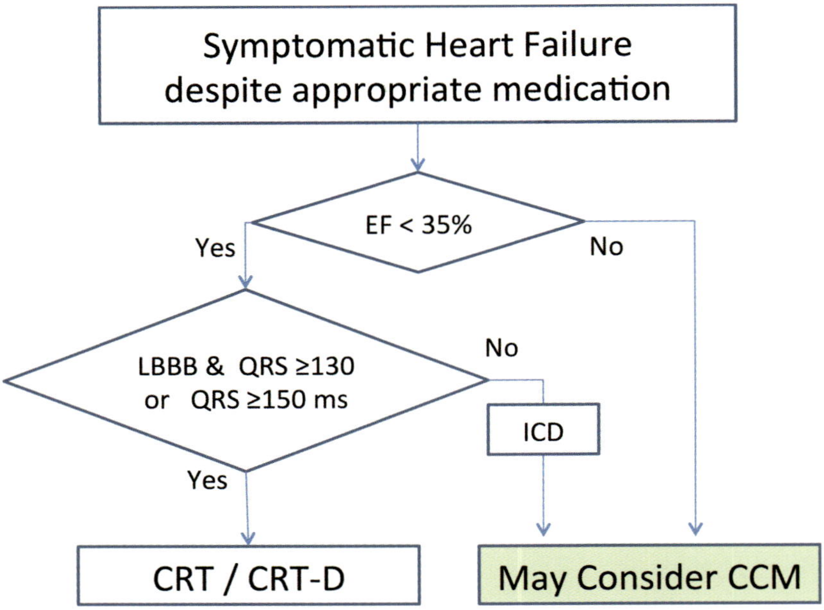

FIGURE 11.1 Patients for whom CRT is indicated and those in whom CCM may be considered

QRS>150 ms and are candidates for CRT[1]. However for the remaining 2/3 of subjects with heart failure and EF<35%, CRT is not indicated or even contraindicated (normal QRS duration).[1,3] In these patients, cardiac contractility modulation (CCM) may be considered as a means to offer symptomatic and functional benefit.

CCM device characteristics

CCM is a novel cardiac stimulation device that delivers two large amplitude (±7V) biphasic electrical pulses to the ventricular septum (Figure 11.2) for between 5 and 12 hours/day. Because the impulses are delivered 30 ms after the onset of the QRS and are of 20 ms duration, they are initiated and completed within the absolute refractory period of heart. Therefore these signals do not evoke depolarizations or alter the underlying cardiac activation sequence. They are not associated with initiation of ventricular arrhythmias. CCM elicits both acute and sustained improvements in contraction with favorable cardiac remodeling and improvement in symptoms and exercise tolerance. The CCM delivery system (OPTIMIZER IV) consists of three implantable commercial leads, one in the right atrium for detecting and timing atrial activation, and two

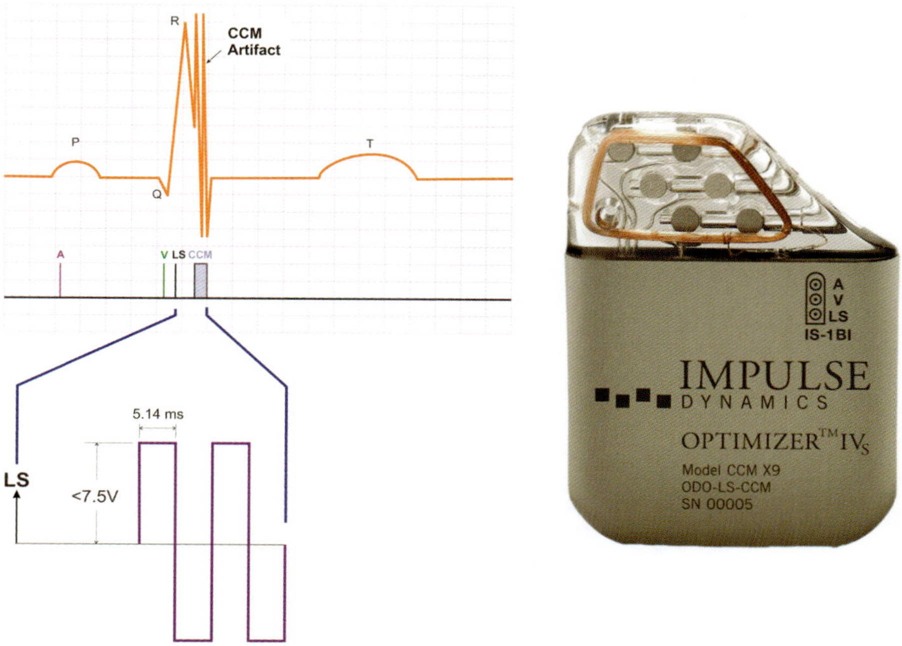

FIGURE 11.2 The Optimizer™ System for Cardiac Contractility Modulation (CCM™) applies non-excitatory signals during the absolute refractory period

bipolar electrodes in the right ventricular septum approximately 2 cm apart for sensing ventricular depolarization and delivering the CCM impulse. Leads are connected to a subcutaneously inserted pulse generator box over the pectoral muscle on the opposite side of the chest from other implanted devices (e.g. ICD). The insertion process is similar to that of a pacemaker. Because of the large current delivered, the pulse generator battery is typically charged weekly with a specialized external conductive magnet.

Effects of CCM on cardiac function and remodeling

Onset of the CCM signal is associated with a rapid increase in isolated myocyte muscle force occurring with the next beat (Figure 11.3a).[4] Offset of the force generation is equally swift. This parallels with the observed rapid increases (within 3–5 minutes) in LV ejection fraction, dP/dt, and stroke volume that are observed in vivo.[5–8] These hemodynamic improvements result in long term structural adaptive remodeling of the failing ventricle (Figure 11.3b).[8,9]

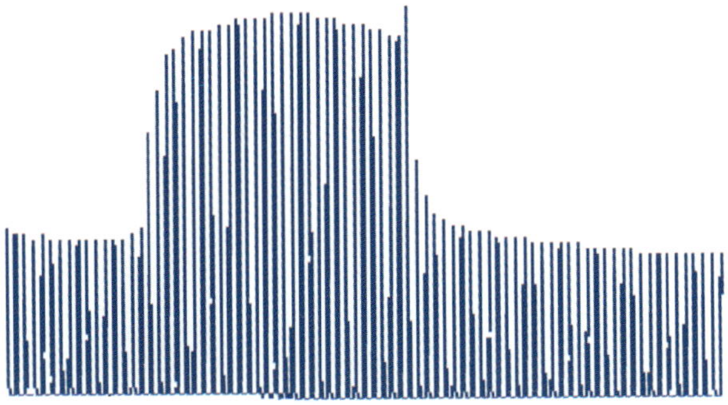

FIGURE 11.3A Acute effect of increased myocardial contractility

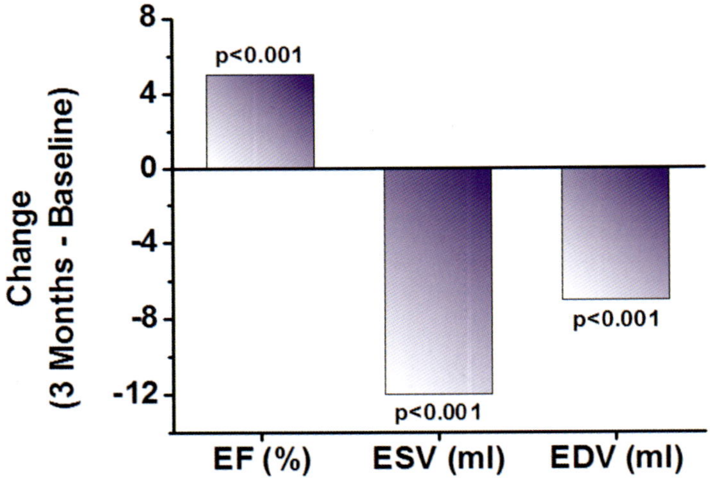

FIGURE 11.3B Functional and structural reverse remodeling[9]

Chronic improvements in cardiac contractility and structure with CCM therapy are accompanied by reversal of the foetal gene programming that occurs with heart failure and by improvement in cardiomyocyte calcium handling. ANP and BNP levels which are elevated in heart failure, are reduced with CCM treatment. Conversely expression of the primary contractile protein, α-myosin heavy chain, which is typically depressed in chronic heart failure, is increased following chronic treatment with CCM.[10,11] Heart failure is also associated with abnormal cardiomyocyte calcium handling. In humans and animals with heart failure, SERCA2a is downregulated, with reductions in phospholamban phosphorylation, reduced ryanodine receptor expression, and an elevation in the sodium-calcium exchanger content.[10] These changes reduce depolarization-induced calcium release thereby attenuating contractility. Chronic application of CCM in heart failure restores these biochemical abnormalities towards normal, thus improving contractile efficiency of the failing myocardium. Interestingly these biochemical changes are first observed in the region where impulse delivery occurs but after a few months of treatment, the beneficial adaptation extends to remote regions of the myocardium as well.[10] Each of these benefits associated with CCM treatment (structural remodeling, reversion away from the foetal gene programming, and biochemical restoration of cardiomyocyte calcium handling drives an improvement in cardiac function. Collectively they are likely responsible for the observed improvement in contractile efficiency described with CCM treatment. In humans and in animal models, CCM is associated with an increase in contractile function without an increase in myocardial oxygen consumption, thus an improvement in cardiac contractile efficiency.[12,13]

Clinical evaluation of CCM therapy in heart failure with reduced ejection fraction

CCM has been evaluated in more than 10 clinical trials and registries, with clinical experience in nearly 3000 patients. Enrollment has focused on patients with symptomatic (NYHA II-IV) heart failure with reduced ejection fraction (typically 35% or less) and without prolonged QRS duration. Results from the three major randomized controlled clinical trials (FIX-HF-4, FIX-HF-5, and FIX-HF-5-pilot)[7,14,15] have been compiled into a meta-analysis based on collective analysis of individual data (Figure 11.4).[2] Exercise tolerance (peak VO_2), walking distance (6 min walk test), and quality of life (Minnesota living with heart failure questionnaire; MLWHFQ) were assessed across 641 individual subjects from the three trials. Compared to controls, those patients with CCM treatment had significantly higher pVO_2 ($p=0.006$) with a better quality of life (MLWHFQ; $p=0.0001$), and a borderline significant improvement in 6MW ($p=0.05$). The magnitude of the overall benefit is only slightly less than what has been published with CRT.[16,17] Safety was also examined and adverse events were not significantly increased in the CCM group. In the largest randomized controlled clinical trial to date there were no differences in serious adverse event rates between OMT and OMT+CCM groups.[7]

A subgroup analysis of FIX-HF-5, planned prior to the start of the trial, suggested a greater benefit of CCM in patients with less severely reduced ejection fractions. When evaluating the 205 subjects from this trial with EF>25%, the primary endpoint (ventilatory aerobic threshold) was significantly improved by

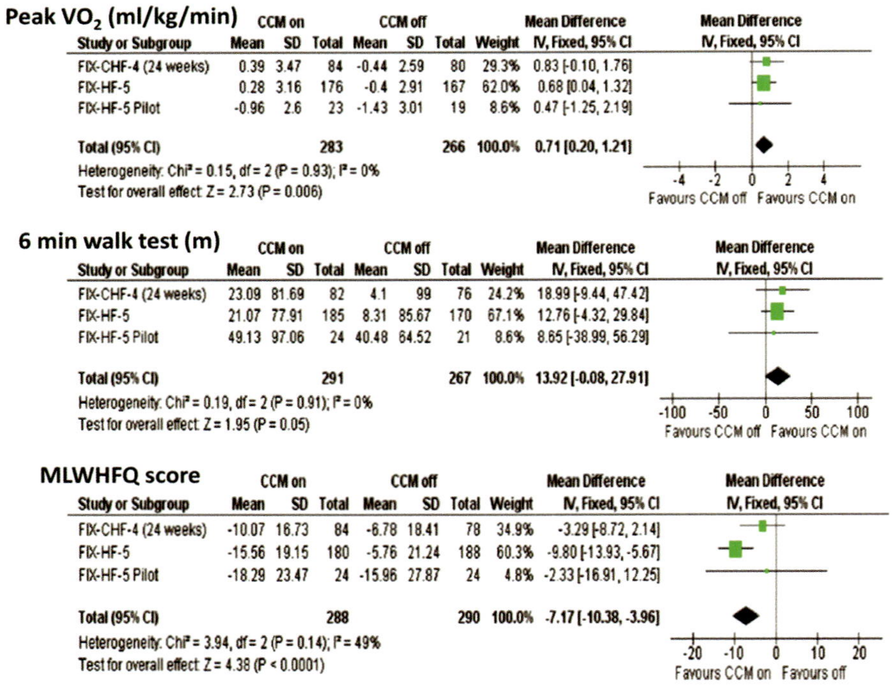

FIGURE 11.4 Individual patient data meta-analysis showing significant improvement in peak VO_2 (top), 6 minute walk distance (middle) and MLWHFQ (lower).[2]

CCM, even though no effect was observed in the total cohort. Improvements in NYHA classification and MLWHFQ were observed in these patients with less severe reductions in ejection fraction (Figure 11.5). When limiting the analysis to those patients with EF>35%, even greater improvements in peak VO_2 and MLWHF were observed (Figure 11.6).[18] A more recent study has also demonstrated a greater benefit of CCM in patients with moderate vs. severe reductions in EF in terms of all-cause mortality and heart failure hospitalizations.[19] These finding support an ongoing controlled randomized clinical trial of CCM+OMT vs. OMT alone in patients with moderately reduced EF (25–45%).[20] They have also prompted the Task Force that developed the 2016 ESC Guidelines for Diagnosis and Treatment of Acute and Chronic Heart Failure to comment on CCM. Although a specific guideline recommendation was not made, the guideline document indicates that in contrast to other novel devices being considered for heart failure, "CCM may be considered in selected patients with HF [heart failure]".[1]

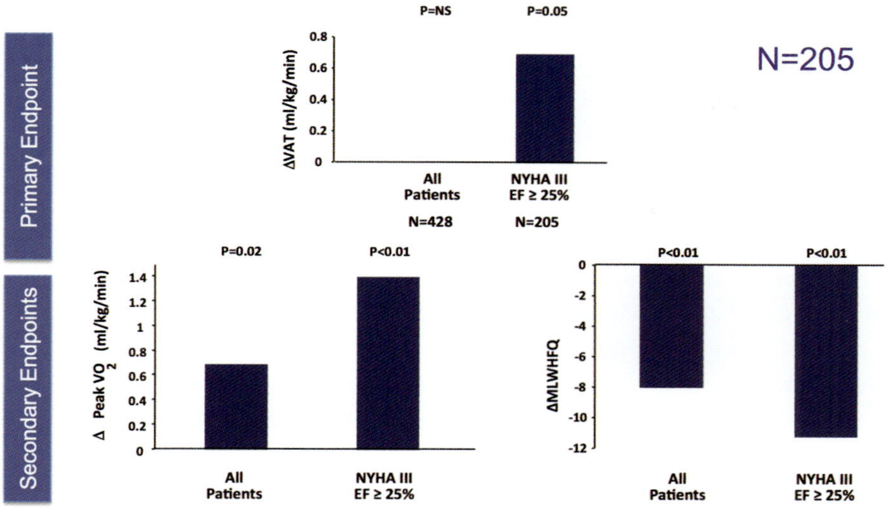

FIGURE 11.5 CCM effects in the patients sub-group with NYHA III and LVEF ≥ 25%[20]

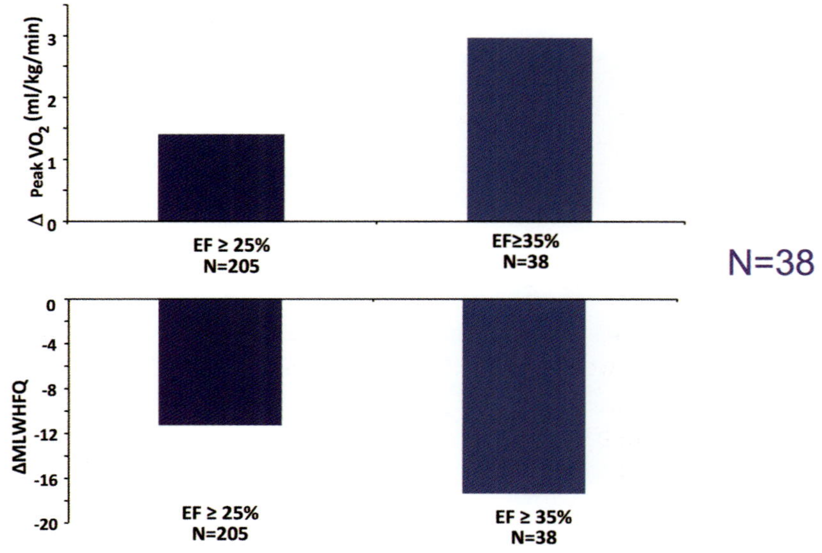

FIGURE 11.6 Larger benefits of CCM in a similar sub-group (NYHA III and LVEF ≥ 35%)[18]

Long term survival analysis

Mortality has not been a primary outcome measure in any of the randomized clinical trials of CCM. However several recent publications document single and multisite experience with patients who have had chronically implanted CCM devices. Schau et al. were first to examine mortality in 54 consecutive patients with NYHA class III-IV heart failure and average EF of 23±6%. Subjects were followed for nearly 3 years and all-cause mortality was compared with mortality in a cohort with similar acuity of disease as predicted by the Seattle Heart Failure Model (SHFM).[22] At the end of 33 months, there was no difference in mortality between the CCM treated group and the SHFM prediction indicating lack of adverse effect of CCM on long-term mortality. Kuschyk and colleagues[23] published long-term follow up in 81 consecutive patients with CCM implantation at a single site. Most patients were NHYA class III and average EF was 23±8%. Survival at 1 and 3 years was better than predicted by the MAGGIC score long term mortality data. Even when correcting for the more frequent use of ICDs in the CCM cohort, mortality rates were no worse than predicted by MAGGIC. A third study was conducted

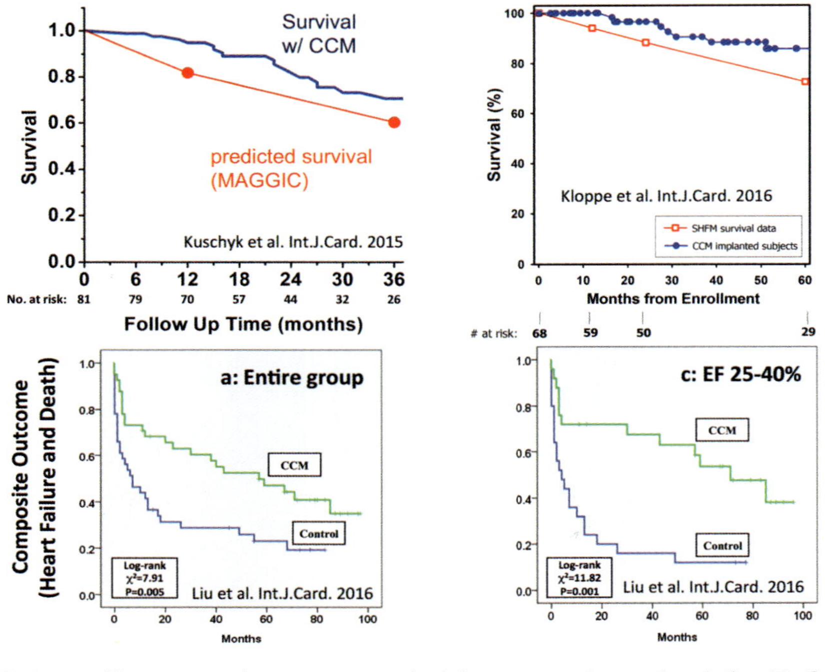

FIGURE 11.7 Reports on long term survival (or composite end-point) with CCM compared to non-randomised matched registry derived data[19,23,24]

across two sites in Germany by Kloppe et al.[24] who followed 68 consecutive patients implanted with CCM. Patients had NYHA class II or III symptoms and EF of 26±6%. Long term mortality was assessed and compared with that predicted by SHFM. Follow up at 1, 2 and 5 years demonstrated a survival with CCM better than predicted by SHFM at each time point. In a recent study with the longest follow-up, Liu et al.[19] examined mortality in 41 consecutively implanted (CCM) patients from a single practice. They compared mortality, hospitalization, and the composite outcome with a contemporaneous control group from a registry of patients in the same practice. Controls were matched for age, gender, EF, and etiology of heart failure. Baseline EF was 27±7% and similar between groups. Outcomes were measured over 5 years (Figure 11.7) and revealed a significant reduction in mortality, hospitalization, and the composite outcome at all time points measured. When patients were stratified according to ejection fraction, the improvement in survival and heart failure hospitalizations was augmented in patients with EF between 25–45% compared to matched controls, but no longer was a difference seen between CCM vs. controls for EF<25%. In a recently presented study that has not yet been

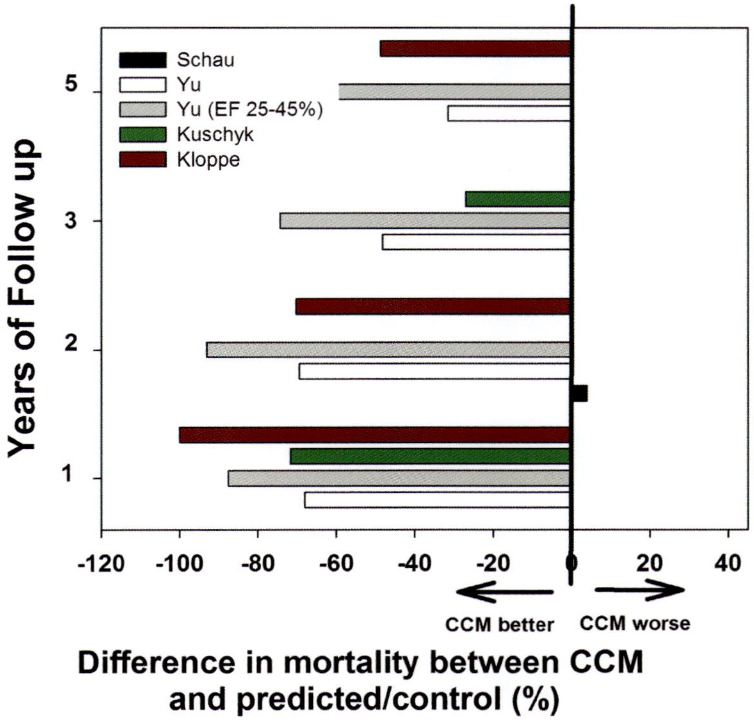

FIGURE 11.8 A composite view of several long term survival reports.[27]

published, Abraham and colleagues determined 3.4 year mortality rates among patients who were implanted with a CCM device as part of their participation in FIX-HF-5. Survival curves were compared to the most contemporary comparator group; namely, patients participating in the PARADIGM-HF study comparing the combination drug Entresto with Lisinopril.[25] Although statistical comparison was not possible between Entresto and CCM, in each group, age, gender, BMI, blood pressure, etiology of HF, and LVEF were similar. The PARADIGM-HF Enalapril group had the highest mortality rate at the 3.5 year study follow up time point, and the FIX-HF-5 subgroup (EF≥25%) had the lowest. Mortality in the PARADIGM-HF entresto cohort was similar to that in the FIX-HF-5 total group.[26] Collectively (see Figure 11.8), these survival studies provide strong support for conducting a prospective randomized controlled survival outcome study of CCM in patients without QRS widening and with moderate reductions in EF.

Conclusion

In summary, CCM is an established treatment in the management of moderate to severely symptomatic heart failure with reduced EF and normal QRS duration. CCM impulse delivery is associated with acute improvements in cardiac contractility. Chronic changes include reversion from fetal to adult gene expression profiles in the heart, improved calcium handling, restorative ventricular remodeling, and improved cardiac function. These changes are responsible for an improvement in efficiency whereby contractility increases without a corresponding increase in oxygen consumption. Randomized controlled clinical trials and their meta-analysis demonstrate improvements in quality of life, exercise capacity, and symptoms of CHF. Multiple provocative retrospective analyses suggest that CCM is associated with a reduction in mortality (especially in those with EF>25%) vs. comparable subjects with heart failure treated by OMT. CCM appears to be most efficacious in that relatively large segment of the heart failure population who have moderate to severe symptoms despite optimal medical therapy, but who do not have prolonged QRS duration or LBBB.

References

1. Ponikowski P, Voors AA, Anker SD, Bueno H, Cleland JG, Coats AJ, Falk V, González-Juanatey JR, Harjola VP, Jankowska EA, Jessup M, Linde C, Nihoyannopoulos P, Parissis JT, Pieske B, Riley JP, Rosano GM, Ruilope LM, Ruschitzka F, Rutten FH, van der Meer P; Authors/Task Force Members; Document Reviewers. 2016 ESC

Guidelines for the diagnosis and treatment of acute and chronic heart failure: The Task Force for the diagnosis and treatment of acute and chronic heart failure of the European Society of Cardiology (ESC) Developed with the special contribution of the Heart Failure Association (HFA) of the ESC. Eur Heart J. 2016 May 20. pii: ehw128. PMID: 27206819.

2. Giallauria F, Vigorito C, Piepoli MF, Stewart Coats AJ. Effects of cardiac contractility modulation by non-excitatory electrical stimulation on exercise capacity and quality of life: An individual patient's data meta-analysis of randomized controlled trials. Int J Cardiol. 2014 Aug 1; 175(2): 352–7. doi:10.1016/j.ijcard.2014.06.005.
3. Shenkman HJ, Pampati V, Khandelwal AK, McKinnon J, et al. Congestive heart failure and QRS duration: establishing prognosis study. Chest. 2002; 122: 528–34.
4. Burkhoff D, Shemer I, Felzen B, Shimizu J, et al. Electric currents applied during the refractory period can modulate cardiac contractility in vitro and in vivo. Heart failure reviews. 2001; 6: 27–34.
5. Lawo T, Borggrefe M, Butter C, Hindricks G, et al. Electrical signals applied during the absolute refractory period: an investigational treatment for advanced heart failure in patients with normal QRS duration. J Am Coll Cardiol. 2005; 46: 2229–36.
6. Pappone C, Rosanio S, Burkhoff D, Mika Y, et al. Cardiac contractility modulation by electric currents applied during the refractory period in patients with heart failure secondary to ischemic or idiopathic dilated cardiomyopathy. The American journal of cardiology. 2002; 90: 1307–13.
7. Kadish A, Nademanee K, Volosin K, Krueger S, et al. A randomized controlled trial evaluating the safety and efficacy of cardiac contractility modulation in advanced heart failure. Am Heart J. 2011; 161: 329–337 e1–2.
8. Morita H, Suzuki G, Haddad W, Mika Y, et al. Long-term effects of non-excitatory cardiac contractility modulation electric signals on the progression of heart failure in dogs. European journal of heart failure. 2004; 6: 145–50.
9. Yu CM, Chan JY, Zhang Q, Yip GW, et al. Impact of cardiac contractility modulation on left ventricular global and regional function and remodeling. JACC Cardiovascular imaging. 2009; 2: 1341–9.
10. Imai M, Rastogi S, Gupta RC, Mishra S, et al. Therapy with cardiac contractility modulation electrical signals improves left ventricular function and remodeling in dogs with chronic heart failure. J Am Coll Cardiol. 2007; 49: 2120–8.
11. Butter C, Rastogi S, Minden HH, Meyhofer J, et al. Cardiac contractility modulation electrical signals improve myocardial gene expression in patients with heart failure. J Am Coll Cardiol. 2008; 51: 1784–9.
12. Goliasch G, Khorsand A, Schutz M, Karanikas G, et al. The effect of device-based cardiac contractility modulation therapy on myocardial efficiency and oxidative metabolism in patients with heart failure. European journal of nuclear medicine and molecular imaging. 2011; 39: 408–15.
13. Butter C, Wellnhofer E, Schlegl M, Winbeck G, et al. Enhanced inotropic state of the failing left ventricle by cardiac contractility modulation electrical signals is not associated with increased myocardial oxygen consumption. J Card Fail. 2007; 13: 137–42.
14. Borggrefe MM, Lawo T, Butter C, Schmidinger H, et al. Randomized, double blind

study of non-excitatory, cardiac contractility modulation electrical impulses for symptomatic heart failure. Eur Heart J. 2008; 29: 1019–28.

15. Neelagaru SB, Sanchez JE, Lau SK, Greenberg SM, et al. Nonexcitatory, cardiac contractility modulation electrical impulses: feasibility study for advanced heart failure in patients with normal QRS duration. Heart rhythm : the official journal of the Heart Rhythm Society. 2006; 3: 1140–7.
16. Cazeau S, Leclercq C, Lavergne T, Walker S, et al. Effects of multisite biventricular pacing in patients with heart failure and intraventricular conduction delay. N Engl J Med. 2001; 344: 873–80.
17. Abraham WT, Fisher WG, Smith AL, DeLurgio DB, et al. Cardiac resynchronization in chronic heart failure. NEnglJMed. 2002; 346: 1845–1853.
18. Borggrefe M and Burkhoff D. Clinical effects of cardiac contractility modulation (CCM) as a treatment for chronic heart failure. European journal of heart failure. 2012; 14: 703–12.
19. Liu M, Fang F, Luo XX, Shlomo BH, et al. Improvement of long-term survival by cardiac contractility modulation in heart failure patients: A case-control study. International journal of cardiology. 2016; 206: 122–6.
20. Abraham WT, Nademanee K, Volosin K, et al. Subgroup analysis of a randomized controlled trial evaluating the safety and efficacy of cardiac contractility modulation in advanced heart failure. J Card Fail. 2011 Sep; 17(9): 710–7. doi:10.1016/j.cardfail.2011.05.006.
21. Abraham WT, Lindenfeld J, Reddy VY, Hasenfuss G, et al. A randomized controlled trial to evaluate the safety and efficacy of cardiac contractility modulation in patients with moderately reduced left ventricular ejection fraction and a narrow QRS duration: study rationale and design. J Card Fail. 2015; 21: 16–23.
22. Schau T, Seifert M, Meyhofer J, Neuss M, et al. Long-term outcome of cardiac contractility modulation in patients with severe congestive heart failure. Europace : European pacing, arrhythmias, and cardiac electrophysiology : journal of the working groups on cardiac pacing, arrhythmias, and cardiac cellular electrophysiology of the European Society of Cardiology. 2011; 13: 1436–44.
23. Kuschyk J, Roeger S, Schneider R, Streitner F, et al. Efficacy and survival in patients with cardiac contractility modulation: long-term single center experience in 81 patients. International journal of cardiology. 2015; 183: 76–81.
24. Kloppe A, Lawo T, Mijic D, Schiedat F, et al. Long-term survival with cardiac contractility modulation in patients with NYHA II or III. International journal of cardiology. 2016.
25. McMurray JJ, Packer M, Desai AS, Gong J, et al. Angiotensin-neprilysin inhibition versus enalapril in heart failure. N Engl J Med. 2014; 371: 993–1004.
26. Abraham WT, Burkhoff D, Rousso B, Morley D, et al. Favorable Long-term Mortality Profile in NYHA III/IV Patients Treated with Contractility Modulation (CCM). 2016.
27. Abi-Samra and Gutterman, Heart Fail Rev. 2016 (in press).

12

The potential of devices for HFpEF

Background

The 2016 ESC/HFA HF guidelines list the very many drug and device therapies that are proven to be beneficial in terms of life prolongation and hospitalisation prevention for HFrEF.[1] The list of recommended therapies or devices for HFpEF and HFmrEF is limited to diuretics and the management of comorbidities and so far there is no clinical evidence for an electrical or mechanical device for HFpEF. The Cardiac Contractility Modulation (CCM) device that may have a role in selected HFrEF and HFmrEF patients has been reviewed in another chapter but here we survey the results so far of a novel device for patients with HFpEF.

Heart failure affects more than 26 million people globally. Heart failure with preserved ejection fraction (HFpEF), accounts for approximately 50% of all heart failure, affecting more than 6.2 million people in the United States and Europe, yet recommended treatment options remain limited. In contrast to the situation of HFrEF the survival risk of HFpEF has virtually remained unchanged over the last two decades of progress in HF research. This is a reflection of the lack of available therapies. Drug treatments for HFpEF and HFmrEF are reviewed in Chapter 7. For HFpEF although prognosis when corrected for age and co-morbidities is lower than for HFrEF it is still unacceptably high. In addition many with this type of heart failure have difficulty breathing, find simple daily activities tiring if not impossible and are frequently hospitalized with a resultant dramatic reduction in their quality of life. Although the pathophysiology of HFpEF is complex and undoubtedly there are several phenotypes of this syndrome it is clear that a sub-set of patients and many of the symptoms are limited by excessive rises in left atrial pressure, in particular during exercise. This is the principal target of left atrial compression with diuretic usage and fluid balance control. The technique of using a device to lower left atrial pressures is novel and offers some potential for the large unmet need of HFpEF patients. Here we review the clinical trials data of one such device, the Corvia Medical IASD®.

The device

Corvia Medical's InterAtrial Shunt Device (IASD) System (Figure 12.1) has derived from pioneering haemodynamic studies going back two decades. The device is a CE-marked investigational, non-surgical transcatheter implant designed to provide continuous and dynamic decompression of the left atrium, in an effort to reduce symptoms, HF hospitalizations, and improve quality of life as well as potentially slowing the progression of HFpEF.

The device is designed to be inserted percutaneously during a catheter-based procedure. The delivery system is used to create a controlled inter-atrial communication, with resulting flow through the IASD system between the left and right atria. This opening allows blood to flow from the high pressure left atrium to the lower pressure right atrium and can decrease the elevated left atrial pressures in HFpEF in a dynamic manner i.e. at rest and during physical activity, thereby reducing lung congestion. Figure 12.2 shows the implant loaded on the delivery catheter.

This device based approach has been developed, in part based upon the observation that patients with Lutembacher's syndrome (ASD + Mitral Stenosis and some congenital heart patients with ASD's) are less symptomatic than those without an ASD, suggesting that left atrial decompression through an inter-atrial communication might relieve symptoms in HFpEF where like in

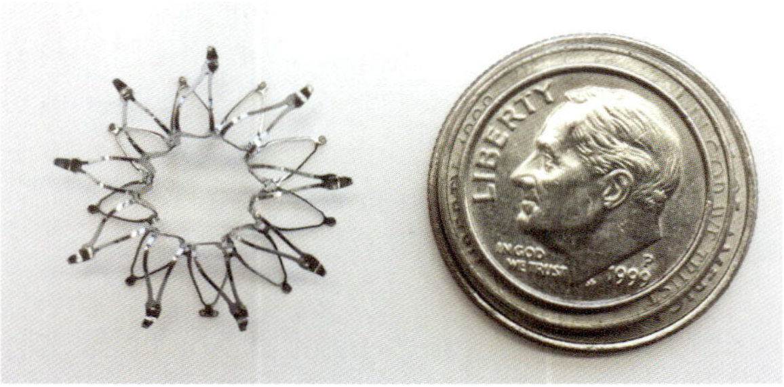

FIGURE 12.1 The Corvia InterAtrial Shunt Device (IASD®) System. The device next to a US 10 cent coin for size comparison.

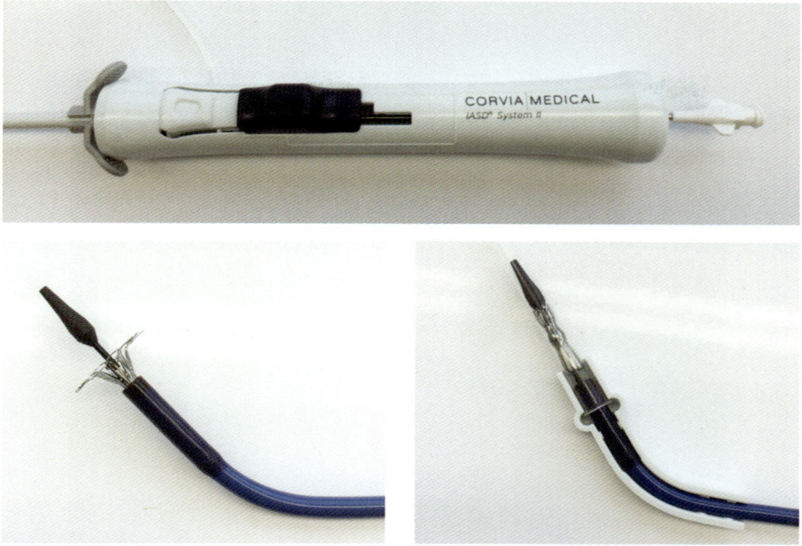

FIGURE 12.2 The IASD delivery system. Panel A shows the controller of the delivery catheter system. Panel B shows the device still loaded onto the catheter delivery system and Panel C shows the device half deployed.

MS left atrial pressures are elevated.[2] This thinking led to the first in man experience in patients initially with MS and subsequently in HFpEF. Simulation modelling showed the theoretical effects of such a shunt (diameter up to 12 mm) on acute rest and exercise haemodynamic data (including changes in PCWP) in patients with HFpEF. The inter-atrial shunt was predicted to lower PCWP acutely by ~3 mm Hg under simulated resting conditions (from 10 to 7 mm Hg) and by ~11 mm Hg during simulated peak exercise (from 28 to 17 mm Hg). Left ventricular cardiac output was predicted to decrease ~0.5 L/min at rest and ~1.3 L/min at peak exercise, with corresponding increases in right ventricular cardiac output. A majority of these effects were achieved with a shunt diameter of 8–9 mm, whereas minimal effects were obtained with diameters under 6 mm.[3]

Based on these data a first pilot study in patients with HFpEF was commenced.[4] Eleven patients satisfying the inclusion/exclusion criteria of symptomatic HFpEF and LVEF >45%; baseline PCWP ≥15 mmHg (at rest), or ≥ 25 mmHg (on exercise) were included. An IASD device was successfully implanted in all 11 using percutaneous trans-septal access via the femoral vein. At 30 days, LV filling pressures had fallen 5.5 mmHg (19.7 ± 3.4 vs. 14.2 ± 2.7; P = 0.005. Two serious adverse events were reported (one re-hospitalization,

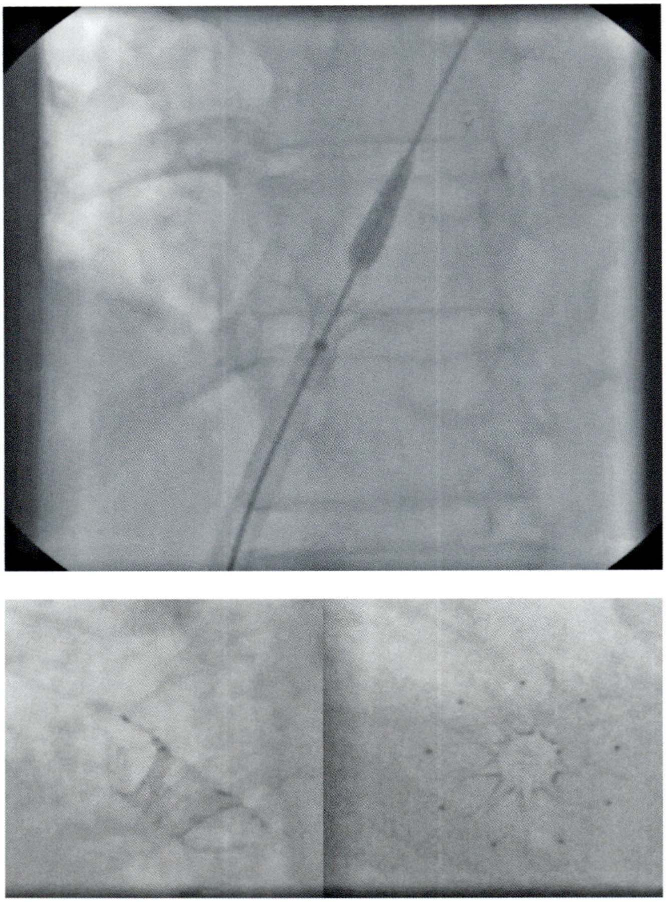

FIGURE 12.3 Panel A: The device being deployed. Panel B: two views of a fully deployed device

and one implant malposition successfully treated with a new device during the index procedure). One of these implantations is shown in Figure 12.3 and the desired placement of the device showed figuratively in Figure 12.4. At one year, all patients had survived, NYHA class had decreased (Class III/IV 45 %/0 % vs. 82%/18% at baseline), six-minute walk distance had increased (315±152 meters to 343±76 meters) and MLWHF score improved (53±17 to 37±17), although these changes were not statistically significant. Over the year compared to the year pre-implantation heart failure hospitalisations decreased from affecting 6 of 11 patients with a rate per 10 patient years of 1.36 to 2 of 11 patients, and a HFH/10PY rate of 0.73. (p=0.03).

Theses encouraging early proof of concept results led to the design of the

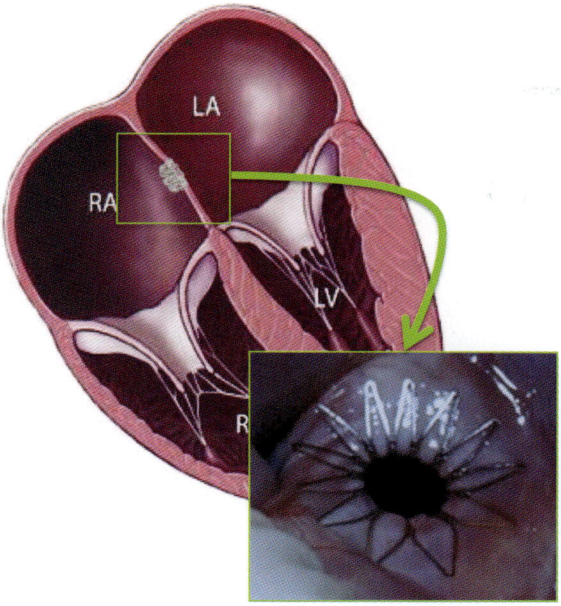

FIGURE 12.4 conceptual picture of placement of the IASD

REDUCE LAP-HF Trial[6] in which patients with ejection fraction ≥40% and New York Heart Association functional class III or IV heart failure with a pulmonary pressure (PCWP) ≥15 mm Hg at rest or ≥25 mm Hg during supine bike exercise were planned to be implanted with an IASD System II, and followed for three years. This trial has recently reported[7] and showed in 68 HFpEF patients (placement successful in 64 of 66) no major adverse cardiac or cerebrovascular events through 6 months. At 6 months, 31 (52%) of 60 patients had a reduction in pulmonary capillary wedge pressure at rest and 34 (58%) of 59 had a lower pulmonary capillary wedge pressure during exertion, with 39% achieving both. Exercise wedge pressure was reduced both at 20 watts (–3 mmHg, p=0·0124) and at peak exercise (–2 mmHg, p=0·0255), despite an improved exercise duration (7·3 min [SD 3·1] vs 8·2 min [3·4], p=0·03). Sustained device patency at 6 months was confirmed by left-to-right shunting (pulmonary/systemic flow ratio: 1·06 [SD 0·32] at baseline vs 1·27 [0·20] at 6 months, p=0·0004).

Conclusions

Despite lagging many years behind HFrEF, HFpEF patients are now being targeted with novel devices with the potential to improve symptoms, improve quality of life, reduce hospitalization and delay progression of the syndrome. The front-runner is a novel inter-atrial left atrial pressure decompression device the Corvia IASD, currently enrolling patients in a randomized trial.

References

1. Ponikowski P, Voors A, Anker S et al The Task Force for the diagnosis and treatment of acute and chronic heart failure of the European Society of Cardiology (ESC). 2016 ESC Guidelines for the diagnosis and treatment of acute and chronic heart failure. European Journal of Heart Failure. Published online 26 May 2016.
2. Kaye D, Malek F, Gustafsson F, et al. Initial Six Month Results of a Novel Inter-atrial Shunt Therapy for Heart Failure with Preserved Ejection Fraction. Presented at ACC 2014.
3. Kaye D, Shah SJ, Borlaug BA, Gustafsson F, Komtebedde J, Kubo S, Magnin C, Maurer MS, Feldman T, Burkhoff D. Effects of an interatrial shunt on rest and exercise hemodynamics: results of a computer simulation in heart failure. J Card Fail. 2014 Mar; 20(3): 212–21. doi:10.1016/j.cardfail.2014.01.005.
4. Søndergaard L, Reddy V, Kaye D, et al. Transcatheter Treatment of Heart Failure with Preserved or Mildly Reduced Ejection Fraction Using a Novel Interatrial Implant to Lower Left Atrial Pressure. Eur J Heart Failure 2014; 16: 796–801.
5. Malek F, Neuzil P, Gustafsson F, et al. Clinical Outcome of Transcatheter Treatment of Heart Failure with Preserved or Mildly Reduced Ejection Fraction Using a Novel Implant. International Journal of Cardiology 2015; 187: 227–28.
6. Hasenfuβ G, Gustafsson F, Kaye D, et al. Rationale and Design of the Reduce Elevated Left Atrial Pressure in Patients With Heart Failure (Reduce LAP-HF) Trial. J Card Fail 2015; 21(7): 594–600.
7. Hasenfuß G, Hayward C, Burkhoff D, et al. A transcatheter intracardiac shunt device for heart failure with preserved ejection fraction (REDUCE LAP-HF): a multicentre, open-label, single-arm, phase 1 trial. Lancet. 2016 Mar 26; 387(10025): 1298–304. doi:10.1016/S0140-6736(16)00704-2.
8. Feldman T, Komtebedde J, Burkhoff D, et al. Transcatheter Interatrial Shunt Device for the Treatment of Heart Failure: Rationale and Design of the Randomized Trial to REDUCE Elevated Left Atrial Pressure in Heart Failure (REDUCE LAP-HF I) Circ. Heart Fail. 2016; 9: e003025. doi:10.1161/CIRCHEARTFAILURE.116.003025.

13

The management of diabetic patients with heart failure

Introduction

Patients with diabetes mellitus have an increased risk of developing heart failure and diabetes mellitus is highly prevalent amongst patients with heart failure, especially those with HFpEF.[1–3] Diabetic patients with heart failure have an increased mortality and an increased risk of hospitalisations and the use of certain anti-diabetic agents increase the risk of mortality and hospitalisation in heart failure.[4] Conversely, newer therapeutic agents have shown a significant reduction of mortality, morbidity and risk of developing heart failure in diabetic patients with proven cardiovascular disease.[5]

Epidemiological evidence clearly shows that diabetes mellitus is independently associated with the risk of developing HF. This risk increases by more than two-folds in men and by five-fold in women.[6] In patients with diabetes mellitus the prevalence of HF is reported to be up to 25%, which is 4 times higher than that observed in the general population. The prevalence of diabetes mellitus is even higher in acute heart failure where it reaches 40%. The complex relationship between diabetes mellitus and heart failure is shown by the fact that patients with heart failure and without diabetes have an increased risk of developing heart failure diabetes compared to a matched population (29% vs 18% respectively).[1–3,6]

A meta-analysis of 21 studies including 1,111,569 patients including 507,637 with diabetes mellitus showed that age, diabetes duration, insulin use, ischaemic heart disease, and elevated serum creatinine are independent risk factors for the development of heart failure in diabetics.[7] The relationship between diabetes mellitus and heart failure is not just the result of the sum

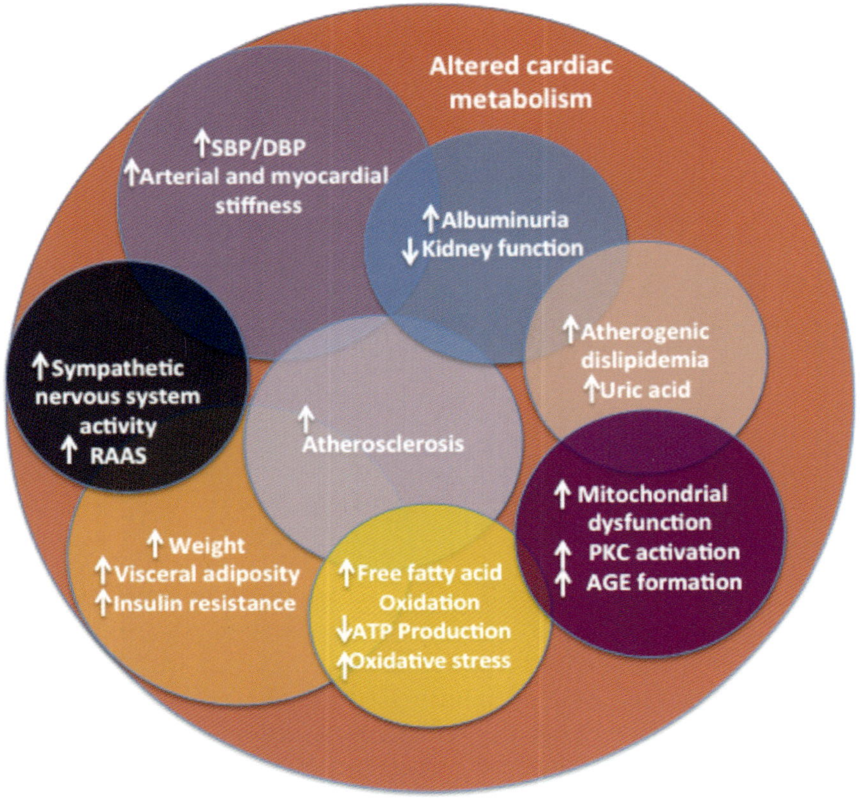

FIGURE 13.1 Diabetes related mechanism for the development of HF

of the parts since each condition adversely affects the natural course of the other and results in a poorer prognosis than with either disease alone. Since heart failure has a much poorer prognosis than diabetes mellitus is has to be a priority for treatment in patients presenting with the two morbidities.

Altered glucose metabolism of patients with impaired glucose control and diabetes mellitus contribute to structural and functional abnormalities of the heart, culminating in cardiac dysfunction and ultimately CHF, not only via coronary artery disease (CAD), for which altered glucose metabolism is a major and independent risk factor, but also via other multiple pathophysiologic and metabolic abnormalities.[8] Impaired cardiac glucose metabolism has a significant negative effect on cardiac contractility and functioning thereby inducing left ventricular systolic and diastolic dysfunction even in absence of CAD or structural heart disease.[9–10]

Hyperglycemia and insulin resistance also contribute to the development of heart failure through several different mechanisms acting independently and synergistically such as impaired microvascular endothelial function, abnormal cardiac metabolism (shift myocardial utilization of glucose toward less efficient fatty acid oxidation), increased myocardial fibrosis, increased oxidative stress and local activation of the renin-angiotensin system and sympathetic nervous system.[9–10]

The SOLVD trial showed that diabetic patients had higher all cause and cardiovascular mortality compared to non-diabetic patients. Subsequently, both population studies and clinical trials have demonstrated that diabetes mellitus significantly increases the risk of recurrent HF hospitalizations and hospital stay in patients with heart failure and it is associated with a significantly higher mortality compared to those without diabetes.[11]

Diabetes mellitus was the most relevant co-morbidity affecting prognosis of patients with heart failure in the Candesartan in Heart failure—Assessment of Reduction in Mortality and morbidity (CHARM) program. In this study the presence of diabetes mellitus was associated with an approximate 2-fold increase of either death or the composite outcome of cardiovascular death or hospitalization for heart failure in insulin users, and a 50% increase risk in non insulin-treated diabetics.[3]

The increased mortality rate of diabetic patients with heart failure is observed in both patients with reduced and preserved left ventricular ejection fraction as well as in patients with heart failure due to either ischaemic or non-ischaemic origin. However, the interaction between diabetes mellitus and outcomes is weaker in hospitalized patient for acute heart failure suggesting that in hospitalized patients the prognosis depends more on the severity of HF de-compensation rather than on the presence of co-morbidities.

While the efficacy and safety of the cardiovascular drugs for the treatment of heart failure in diabetic patients are well known those of glucose lowering therapies is uncertain, potentially harmful and not adequately evaluated for most drug classes.[4] Also, the adequate level of glucose control in diabetic patients with heart failure is under debate but higher levels of HbA1c should be recommended for diabetic patients with heart failure.[12]

Treatment of heart failure in patients with diabetes

No randomised clinical trials have been specifically performed to study the effects of pharmacological and non-pharmacological interventions in diabetic patients with heart failure. However, a wealth of evidence suggests that all interventions that improve prognosis in patients with heart failure are equally beneficial in patients with and without diabetes.[12]

This evidence comes from robust subgroup analyses of the large randomised controlled trials conducted in patients with heart failure in which usually at least 30% of diabetic patients have been enrolled. Beta-blockers and Angiotensin-converting Enzyme Inhibitors are beneficial in patients with diabetes and their use is associated with reduced mortality and hospitalisations. Angiotensin II receptor blockers have shown similar efficacy in heart failure patients with and without diabetes. Although non-selective beta blockers may have a negative affect on glycaemic control and increase the risk of future diabetes, these effects should be less frequent with the more selective agents such as bisoprolol, carvedilol and nebivolol. There is no reason from the major trials, however, to suggest a preferential use of a beta blocker over another on the basis of the possible negative effect on glucose control. Despite these findings, diabetic patients are still less likely to be discharged from hospital on a β-blocker than non-diabetic patients with HF.[12]

Mineralocorticoid receptor antagonists reduce the risk of hospitalization and premature death and they are equally effective in patients with heart failure with and without diabetes mellitus. Because of the frequent occurrence of diabetic nephropathy the possibility of hyperkalaemia should always be considered and a close surveillance of electrolyte and renal function is recommended. LCZ696, and Ivabradine have been shown to be similarly effective in heart failure patients with and without diabetes and should be implemented as appropriate.[12]

Glucose lowering treatment in patients with diabetes and HF

The relevance of glucose lowering agents in patients with heart failure or at increased risk of heart failure has become evident after Rosiglitazone, a thiazolidinezone, was withdrawn from the EU and the USA market because of the evidence of increased risk of cardiovascular events.[13] Although, most of the meta-analyses and the regulatory agencies focused mainly on the risk of coronary events, it was evident that the most significant risk with the use of this drug(s) was related to heart failure.

There are several pathophysiological reasons because a glucose-lowering agent may favour the development of heart failure. These relate to the increased insulin levels, water retention and low glucose availability for the heart and muscles.

One important point in diabetic patients with heart failure but relevant to all patients with dys-glycaemia is the target level of glycated haemoglobin that should be regarded as optimal. From the publication of the UKPDS study onwards almost all studies targeting HbA1c levels <7.5% failed to show a cardiovascular benefit and often demonstrated an increased risk of cardiovascular mortality and morbidity, most often related to heart failure.[1,14–18] In patients with heart failure and co-existing diabetes mellitus maintenance of adequate glycaemic control is a critical issue not only because of the relationship between glucose levels, heart function and outcomes but also because the choice of drugs available to safely manage glucose management in patients with heart failure is limited.[8,9]

A meta-analysis of 13 high quality studies on 34,533 patients showed that intensive glucose lowering is not associated with any significant reduction in cardiovascular risk but conversely results in a 47% increase in HF risk ($P<0.001$).[19] More recently, a study conducted in a large cohort of heart failure patients with T2DM showed a U-shaped relationship between HbA1c and mortality, with the lowest risk in patients with moderate glycaemic control (HbA1c 7.1–8.0%) and those treated with insulin sensitizers. Of interest the U-shaped relationship between glucose control and events seems to be present in drug-treated but not in diet-treated diabetic patients.[14]

These findings concur with the results of the ACCORD study, which demonstrated that very tight control of glucose in patients with diabetes mellitus increases by 22% the risk of death from all causes and by 35% the occurrence of cardiovascular death.[20] The Eplerenone Post-Acute Myocardial Infarction Heart Failure Efficacy and Survival Study (EPHESUS) also found a 38% increased risk of a poorer outcome among patients with hypoglycaemia complicating HF post-MI.[21] In diabetic patients with heart failure a clear difference in the occurrence of adverse outcomes seems also to be related to the type of anti-diabetic medications as patients on drugs with a low risk of hypoglycaemia seem to have a better prognosis than those on medications known to be associated with a high risk of hypoglycaemia risk (secretagogues or insulin).[4,14]

Treatment of diabetes in patients with heart failure

The treatment of elevated glucose plasma levels should be carefully evaluated and gradually implemented in diabetic patients with heart failure. In the early stages of diabetes mellitus and throughout patient life preference should be given to metformin that has been shown to be safe and effective.[22,23] Since metformin is excreted though the kidney caution should be exerted in patients with impaired renal function while its use is contraindicated only in patients with severe renal or hepatic impairment. As mentioned above, sulphonylurea derivatives may more frequently induce hypoglycaemia, although this risk is minimised by slow release formulations. An increased risk of worsening heart failure has been reported with sulphonylureas in diabetic patients but has never been proven in prospective randomised clinical trials.[4] Therefore, sulphonylureas should be used with caution in diabetic patients with heart failure.[12]

Metiglinides have a mechanism of action similar to that of sulphonylureas as they bind to an ATP-dependent K+ channel on the membrane of pancreatic beta cells, albeit with a weaker affinity. Because of their effect on insulin secretion, these drugs may induce water retention and should be used with caution in patients with heart failure.

Alpha glucosidase-inhibitors, such as acarbose, inhibit the intestinal alpha glucosidase, an enzyme that releases glucose from larger carbohydrates. Acarbose reduces the rate of digestion of complex carbohydrates and therefore the absorption of glucose, because the carbohydrates are not broken down into glucose molecules. Given the lack of any effect on insulin and water and Na retention, Acarbose is safe to use in patients with increased cardiovascular risk and in those with heart failure.

Thiazolidinediones are a class of drugs that act by activating PPARs (peroxisome proliferator-activated receptors), a group of nuclear receptors, with greatest specificity for PPARγ. These drugs increase the transcription of a number of specific genes and decrease that of others. Their main effect of is a decrease in the amount of free fatty acids present in circulation associated with an increase in the storage of fatty acids in adipocytes and an increased oxidation of carbohydrates. These drugs are associated with an increased fluid retention that results from a reduction in renal excretion of sodium. Furthermore, Thiazolidinediones increase sympathetic nervous system activity, that increases the risk of events in patients with heart failure. Indeed, randomised clinical trials and meta-analyses have shown that Thiazolidinediones increase the risk of heart failure worsening and hospitalisations from heart failure and they are contraindicated in patients with heart failure.[13]

Dipeptidylpeptidase-4 inhibitors (DPP4is; gliptins) and glucagon-like peptide 1 (GLP-1) receptor agonists, are popular drugs for the control of glycaemia in patients with diabetes and they are widely used despite their effect on HbA1c being relatively modest. These drugs increase incretin secretion (DPP4i) or act as incretin mimetics, thereby improving glycaemic indices. Studies with DPP4i's have casted doubts about their safety in heart failure since earlier studies have shown an increased risk of heart failure in diabetic patients.[24,25] More recent data suggest that they may be safe to use but given their limited clinical benefit and given that there is a lack of data on their effect in patients with heart failure, their use is not recommended except under strict cardiology supervision.[12,26]

Scanty data exist on the long-term safety of GLP1 receptor agonists and no data in patients with heart failure are available. Recently Liraglutide was studied against placebo in the LEADER trial for a period of up to 5 years in more than 9,000 adults with type 2 diabetes at high cardiovascular risk. The trial showed that liraglutide treatment led to a significant reduction in the composite primary outcome of the first occurrence of cardiovascular death, non-fatal myocardial infarction or non-fatal stroke. Given the absence of detailed data in patients with heart failure, the use of liraglutide (as of all GLP1 receptor agonists) should be implemented only under strict cardiology supervision.

The sodium/glucose co-transporter 2 inhibitors (SGLT2i) enhance glucose control by increasing the urinary excretion of glucose. Recently, the SGLT2i empagliflozin showed a significant and relevant effect on cardiovascular protection.[27] The EMPA-REG OUTCOME study conducted in 7020 patients with type 2 diabetes (glycated hemoglobin level, 7.0 to 10.0%) and at high risk for cardiovascular events and followed for a median of 3.1 years has shown that empagliflozin use led to a significant reduction in the rates of death from cardiovascular causes (38% relative risk reduction), hospitalization for heart failure (35% relative risk reduction), and death from any cause (32% relative reduction). Consistent effects of empagliflozin were observed across all pre-defined subgroups including patients with and without heart failure. A consistent effect of empagliflozin was observed across all drug classes used for the treatment of diabetes and/or heart failure. Of notable importance for patients with heart failure, empagliflozin reduced by 39% the rate of hospitalizations for, or death from heart failure [2.8 vs. 4.5%; HR: 0.61 (0.47–0.79); P < 0.001] and was associated with a reduction in all-cause hospitalization [36.8 vs. 39.6%; HR: 0.89 (0.82–0.96); P = 0.003].

Empagliflozin is the first glucose-lowering agent that had been shown to improve heart failure outcomes in patients with type 2 diabetes and in diabetic patients with heart failure. The mechanisms responsible for the effects of empagliflozin on cardiovascular end-points and heart failure are largely unknown. Potential mechanisms to be proven include an effect on sodium retention and plasma volume, osmotic diuresis, reduction of insulin levels and insulin response to food intake, modulation of the renin angiotensin aldosterone system, reduction in body weight and blood pressure without increases in sympathetic nervous activity. It is possible that the effect of empagliflozin are shared by the drugs in the same class. However, given the recent reports of non-cardiac adverse events with other SGLT2i that had not been observed with empagliflozin and, in the absence of evidence with drugs with similar mechanism of action, the results obtained with empaglifozin cannot be translated to the class of SGLT2i's.

The safety of the different oral hypoglycaemic options in diabetic HF patients is summarised in Table 13.1.

TABLE 13.1 Safety of glucose-lowering treatments for patients with heart failure

Drug	Indication in patients with heart failure
Metformin	Safe to use, first line indication, caution in kidney failure
Sulphonylureas	Use with caution, slow release formulations may induce hypoglycaemia
Thiazolidinediones	Contraindicated
Alpha glucosidase inhibitors	Safe to use
Metiglinides	Use with caution, may induce water retention
Dipeptidylpeptidase-4 inhibitors	Not recommended, use under supervision of the heart failure team
Glucagon-like peptide 1 receptor agonists	Use under supervision of the heart failure team
Sodium/glucose co-transporter 2 inhibitors	Safe to use in diabetic patients Empagliflozin reduces mortality and hospitalisation for heart failure.
Insulin	Use with caution, any change in dose, schedule of administration and type of insulin must be constantly supervised by the heart failure team

Insulin is often required for the glucose control of diabetic patients with type 1 diabetes and of some patients with type 2 diabetes and pancreatic islet beta-cell exhaustion. Since insulin induces significant sodium-retention it can precipitate worsening of heart failure. Although, insulin use in acute patients with heart failure seems safe, in long-term treatment changes in dose, scheduling of administration and the type of insulin used should be constantly supervised by a cardiologist in patients with chronic heart failure to avoid adverse HF-related outcomes. Therefore, the heart failure team according to the clinical conditions should be involved in decisions on the intensity of glycaemic control, the type and dose of glucose lowering agents and any change in the glucose lowering therapy should be closely monitored.

References

1. Stratton IM, Adler AI, Neil HA, Matthews DR, Manley SE, Cull CA, Hadden D, Turner RC, Holman RR. Association of glycaemia with macrovascular and microvascular complications of type 2 diabetes (UKPDS 35): prospective observational study. BMJ 2000; 321: 405–412.
2. Metra M, Zacà V, Parati G, et al. Cardiovascular and noncardiovascular comorbidities in patients with chronic heart failure. Heart Failure Study Group of the Italian Society of Cardiology. J Cardiovasc Med (Hagerstown) 2011; 12: 76–84.
3. MacDonald MR, Petrie MC, Varyani F, et al. Impact of diabetes on outcomes in patients with low and preserved ejection fraction heart failure: an analysis of the Candesartan in Heart failure: Assessment of Reduction in Mortality and morbidity (CHARM) programme. Eur Heart J 2008; 29: 1377–85.
4. Fadini GP, Avogaro A, Degli Esposti L, Russo P, Saragoni S, Buda S, Rosano G, Pecorelli S, Pani L; OsMed Health-DB Network. Risk of hospitalization for heart failure in patients with type 2 diabetes newly treated with DPP-4 inhibitors or other oral glucose-lowering medications: a retrospective registry study on 127,555 patients from the Nationwide OsMed Health-DB Database. Eur Heart J. 2015 Sep 21; 36(36): 2454–62.
5. Zinman B, Wanner C, Lachin JM, Fitchett D, Bluhmki E, Hantel S, et al.Empagliflozin, cardiovascular outcomes, and mortality in type 2 diabetes. N Engl J Med 2015; 373: 2117–28.
6. Ryden L, Grant PJ, Anker SD, Berne C, Cosentino F, Danchin N, et al.ESC Guidelines on diabetes, pre-diabetes, and cardiovascular diseases developed in collaboration with the EASD: the Task Force on diabetes,pre-diabetes, and cardiovascular diseases of the European Society ofCardiology (ESC) and developed in collaboration with the EuropeanAssociation for the Study of Diabetes (EASD). Eur Heart J 2013; 34: 3035–87.
7. Wang Y, Negishi T, Negishi K, Marwick TH. Prediction of heart failure in patients with type 2 diabetes mellitusa systematic review and meta-analysis. Diabetes Res Clin Pract. 2015 Apr; 108(1): 55–66.
8. Rosano GM, Vitale C, Fragasso G. Metabolic therapy for patients with diabetes mellitus and coronary artery disease. Am J Cardiol. 2006 Sep 4; 98(5A): 14J–18J. Epub 2006 Jul 24.
9. Nagoshi T, Yoshimura M, Rosano GM, Lopaschuk GD, Mochizuki S. Optimization of cardiac metabolism in heart failure. Curr Pharm Des. 2011 Dec; 17(35): 3846–53.
10. Rosano GM, Barbaro G. Metabolic therapy: an important therapeutic option for the treatment of cardiovascular diseases. Curr Pharm Des. 2008; 14(25): 2519–20.
11. SOLVD Investigattors. Effect of enalapril on survival in patients with reduced left ventricular ejection fractions and congestive heart failure. N Engl J Med 1991; 325: 293–302.
12. Ponikowski P, Voors A, Anker S et al The Task Force for the diagnosis and treatment of acute and chronic heart failure of the European Society of Cardiology (ESC). 2016 ESC Guidelines for the diagnosis and treatment of acute and chronic heart failure. European Journal of Heart Failure. Published online 26 May 2016.

13. Home PD, Pocock SJ, Beck-Nielsen H, Curtis PS, Gomis R, Hanefeld M, Jones NP, Komajda M, McMurray JJV, for the RECORD Study Team. Rosiglitazone evaluated for cardiovascular outcomes in oral agent combination therapy for type 2 diabetes (RECORD): a multicentre, randomised, open-label trial. Lancet 2009; 373: 2125–35.
14. Elder DHJ, Singh JSS, LevinD, Donnelly LA, Choy AM, George J, Struthers AD, Doney ASF, LangCC. Mean HbA1c and mortality in diabetic individuals with heart failure: a population cohort study. European Journal of Heart Failure (2016) 18, 94–102.
15. Goode KM, John J, Rigby AS, Kilpatrick ES, Atkin SL, Bragadeesh T, Clark AL, Cleland JG. Elevated glycated haemoglobin is a strong predictor of mortality in patients with left ventricular systolic dysfunction who are not receiving treatment for diabetes mellitus. Heart 2009; 95: 917–923.
16. Aguilar D, Bozkurt B, Ramasubbu K, Deswal A. Relationship of haemoglobin A1C and mortality in heart failure patients with diabetes. J Am Coll Cardiol 2009; 54: 422–428.
17. Jeffcoate SL. Diabetes control and complications: the role of glycated haemoglobin, 25 years on. Diabet Med 2004; 21: 657–665.
18. Lind M, Odén A, Fahlén M, Eliasson B. A systematic review of HbA1c variables used in the study of diabetic complications. Diabetes Metab Synd: Clin Res Rev 2008; 2: 282–293.
19. Boussageon R, Bejan-Angoulvant T, Saadatian-Elahi M, Lafont S, Bergeonneau C, Kassaï B, Erpeldinger S, Wright JM, Gueyffier F, Cornu C. Effect of intensive glucose lowering treatment on all cause mortality, cardiovascular death, and microvascular events in type 2 diabetes: meta-analysis of randomised controlled trials. BMJ. 2011 Jul 26; 343: d4169.
20. ACCORD Study Group, Gerstein HC, Miller ME, Genuth S, Ismail-Beigi F, Buse JB, Goff DC Jr, Probstfield JL, Cushman WC, Ginsberg HN, Bigger JT, Grimm RH Jr, Byington RP, Rosenberg YD, Friedewald WT. Long-term effects of intensive glucose lowering on cardiovascular outcomes. N Engl J Med. 2011 Mar 3; 364(9): 818–28.
21. Ukena C, Dobre D, Mahfoud F, Kindermann I, Lamiral Z, Tala S, Rossignol P, Turgonyi E, Pitt B, Böhm M, Zannad F. Hypo- and hyperglycemia predict outcome in patients with left ventricular dysfunction after acute myocardial infarction: data from EPHESUS. J Card Fail 2012; 18: 439–445.
22. MacDonald MR, Eurich DT, Majumdar SR, Lewsey JD, Bhagra S, Jhund PS, Petrie MC, McMurray JJ V, Petrie JR, McAlister FA. Treatment of type 2 diabetes and outcomes in patients with heart failure: a nested case-control study from the U.K. General Practice Research Database. Diabetes Care 2010; 33: 1213–1218.
23. Boussageon R, Supper I, Bejan-Angoulvant T, Kellou N, Cucherat M, Boissel J-P, Kassai B, Moreau A, Gueyffier F, Cornu C. Reappraisal of metformin efficacy in the treatment of type 2 diabetes: a meta-analysis of randomised controlled trials. PLoS Med 2012; 9:e1001204.
24. Monami M, Dicembrini I, Mannucci E. Dipeptidyl peptidase-4 inhibitors and heart failure: a meta-analysis of randomized clinical trials. Nutr Metab Cardiovasc Dis 2014; 24: 689–697.
25. Savarese G, Perrone-Filardi P, D'Amore C, Vitale C, Trimarco B, Pani L, Rosano GMC. Cardiovascular effects of dipeptidyl peptidase-4 inhibitors in diabetic patients: a meta-analysis. Int J Cardiol 2015; 181: 239–244.

26. Green JB, Bethel MA, Armstrong PW, Buse JB, Engel SS, Garg J, Josse R, Kaufman KD, Koglin J, Korn S, Lachin JM, McGuire DK, Pencina MJ, Standl E, Stein PP, Suryawanshi S, Van de Werf F, Peterson ED, Holman RR; TECOS Study Group. Effect of Sitagliptin on Cardiovascular Outcomes in Type 2 Diabetes. N Engl J Med. 2015 Jul 16; 373(3): 232–42.
27. Zinman B, Wanner C, Lachin JM, Fitchett D, Bluhmki E, Hantel S, Mattheus M, Devins T, Johansen OE, Woerle HJ, Broedl UC, Inzucchi SE; EMPA-REG OUTCOME Investigators. Empagliflozin, Cardiovascular Outcomes, and Mortality in Type 2 Diabetes. N Engl J Med. 2015 Nov 26; 373(22): 2117–28.

14

The management of heart failure in kidney and urinary tract syndromes

Introduction

Kidney dysfunction and other related abnormalities are extremely common in all HF syndromes, both because of the similarity of risk factors and the similarity of demography of the two types of patients but also because of the common renal effects of agents used for the treatment of HF. Important renal syndromes for the HF patient include including chronic kidney disease, acute kidney injury, cardio-renal syndrome, and prostatic obstruction. In HF (all types including HFrEF, HFmrEF and especially HFpEF) chronic kidney disease (CKD) frequently co-exists and almost as frequently complicates the HF management. The two groups of syndromes share many risk factors (diabetes, hypertension, hyperlipidaemia) and often interact to worsen the prognosis of each other in a way that makes the patient with combined HF and renal disease at extremely high risk.[1,2] This common co-morbidity and how to manage it has been recently reviewed in the 2016 ESC/HFA heart failure guidelines.[3]

CKD is usually defined as an eGFR <60 mL/min/1.73 m^2 and/or the presence of albuminuria (high 30–300 or very high >300 mg albumin per 1 g of urine creatinine). There is a lack of an adequate evidence base for determining the best way to manage patients with combined HF and severe CKD for, almost universally, those with severe CKD (eGFR <30 mL/min/1.73 m^2) were excluded from the large HF trials.

Another feature of concern is that even those who are started on appropriate HF medication a subsequent change in renal function (even if it were to later prove to be temporary) is used a reason to reduce dosage or cease mediation entirely. This so-called worsening renal function (WRF) is very commonly used clinically as a reason to reduce medication even if it does not satisfy the accepted diagnostic criteria for this term. WRF should be used to indicate an increase in serum creatinine by >26.5 μmol/L (0.3 mg/dL) and/ or a 25% increase, or a 20% drop in glomerular filtration rate (GFR).[3] These small changes in renal function occur commonly but if repeated could progress underlying CKD.[4] Similar worsening of apparent renal function in the setting of an AHF hospitalization or an acute worsening of (decompensated) HF are not always clinically important if they prove to be short-lived. Effective treatments for AHF with appropriate decongestion, diuresis and relief of symptoms may satisfy such a WRF definition in the short-term but not prove detrimental long-term.[5] More significant and more prolonged worsening of renal function (acute kidney injury, AKI) is not as common in the setting of HF. When present there is an urgent need to review therapy as diuretic therapy combined with other nephrotoxic agents (the antibiotic gentamicin and trimethoprim for example, ACEIs, ARBs, NSAIDs, or high dose IV contrast media). It is important to differentiate short-term versus more prolonged changes in apparent renal function. Short-term mild WRF is common in the clinical course of HF patients, especially during initiation and up-titration of RAAS inhibitor therapy or active decongestion with diuretics. If caused by RAAS inhibitor initiation or up-titration the change may be limited in time and extent and in many cases need not lead to permanent treatment discontinuation and unless the WRF is marked treatment benefit is largely maintained (497).[6] If repeated severe WRF should occur when RAAS inhibitors are used the clinician should look out for renal artery stenosis, fluid balance, adequate perfusion and all concomitant medication. Care is essential for electrolyte balance (see chapter on potassium balance).

Diuretic dosages may need to be increased in poor renal function, noting any resultant change in effective renal function. Renal diuretic resistance is more common with reduced renal reserve. Occasionally combination diuretics are needed, particularly a loop diuretic with a thiazide or with metolazone, but this should only be attempted by expert HF managers and only with very close observation on fluid balance, renal function and electrolyte balance.

Care is needed to avoid over-dosing renally excreted drugs such as digoxin, insulin, and low molecular weight heparin. Digoxin levels in particular should be closely monitored in patients with CKD and reduced doses utilized. Particular care is needed during angiography because of the risk of contrast-induced acute kidney injury (CI-AKI). Patients at risk need close monitoring.

Other treatments are used in this setting, although the evidence for popular protective measures such as n-Acetyl cysteine remains weak.

In the setting of Acute HF, especially if severe, severe AKI may be common. In such cases renal replacement therapy may be needed as a short-term measure. The recommendations made in the recent ESC/HFA guidelines[3] state that ultrafiltration may be considered in the presence of AKI with refractory HF congestion, and if diuretic therapy has failed. Formal renal replacement therapy (including dialysis) should be considered in patients with refractory volume overload not responding to medical care.

In the presence of prostatic obstruction (common in older males with HF) care should be taken concerning drug interactions, for example, alpha-adrenoceptor blockers can cause hypotension, and sodium and water retention, and may not be safe in HFrEF.[3,7,8] If needed 5-alpha reductase inhibitors should be used in preference in all male HF patients.

References

1. Damman K, Valente M E, Voors A, O'Connor CM, Van Veldhuisen DJ, Hillege HL. Renal impairment, worsening renal function, and outcome in patients with heart failure: An updated meta-analysis. Eur Heart J 2014; 35: 455–469.
2. Filippatos G, Farmakis D, Parissis J. Renal dysfunction and heart failure: things are seldom what they seem. Eur Heart J 2014; 35: 416–418.
3. Ponikowski P, Voors AA, Anker SD, Bueno H, Cleland JG, Coats AJ, et al. The Task Force for the diagnosis and treatment of acute and chronic heart failure of the European Society of Cardiology (ESC) Developed with the special contribution of the Heart Failure Association (HFA) of the ESC. Eur Heart J. 2016 May 20. pii: ehw128. PMID: 27206819.
4. Chawla LS, Eggers PW, Star RA, Kimmel PL. Acute Kidney Injury and Chronic Kidney Disease as Interconnected Syndromes. N Engl J Med 2014; 371: 58–66.
5. Damman K, Testani JM. The kidney in heart failure: an update. Eur Heart J 2015; 36: 1437–1444.
6. Clark H, Krum H, Hopper I. Worsening renal function during renin-angiotensin-aldosterone system inhibitor initiation and long-term outcomes in patients with left ventricular systolic dysfunction. Eur J Heart Fail 2014; 16: 41–48.
7. Dorszewski A, Göhmann E, Dors ewski B, Werner GS, Kreuzer H, Figulla HR. Vasodilation by urapidil in the treatment of chronic congestive heart failure in addition to angiotensin-converting enzyme inhibitors is not beneficial: results of a placebo-controlled, double-blind study. J Card Fail 1997; 3: 91–96.
8. The ALLHAT Officers and Coordinators for the ALLHAT Collaborative Research Group. Major Cardiovascular Events in Hypertensive Patients Randomized to Doxazosin vs Chlorthalidone. JAMA J Am Med Assoc 2000; 283: 1967–1975.

15

The management of co-morbidities in patients with heart failure – angina and coronary disease

Introduction

Co-morbidities are particularly relevant in the management of HF as they may confound HF diagnosis, worsen symptomatology, impact quality of life and aggravate the prognosis.[1,2] According to the most recent European Society of Cardiology (ESC) guidelines,[1] treatment of co-morbidities is an essential element of the comprehensive care of HF. Angina and coronary artery disease (CAD), in particular are common disorders associated with HF.[3] The pharmacological management of angina according to the ESC guidelines is shown in Figure 15.1 and specific recommendations are listed in Tables 15.1 and 15.2.

Pharmacological treatment

The recommended first-line therapeutic agent for angina control is a beta blocker, due to its efficacy in reducing the risk of HF hospitalisation and the risk of death.[4–7] In appropriately selected HF patients with reduced ejection fraction (HFrEF) angina relief may be obtained with ivabradine as demonstrated by the Systolic Heart failure treatment with the I(f) inhibitor ivabradine Trial (SHIFT).[8] Beta-blockers and ivabradine may also be used to relieve angina symptoms in HF patients with preserved ejection fraction (HFpEF) but further studies are needed.[1]

The addition of trimetazidine to beta-blockers has been also found to

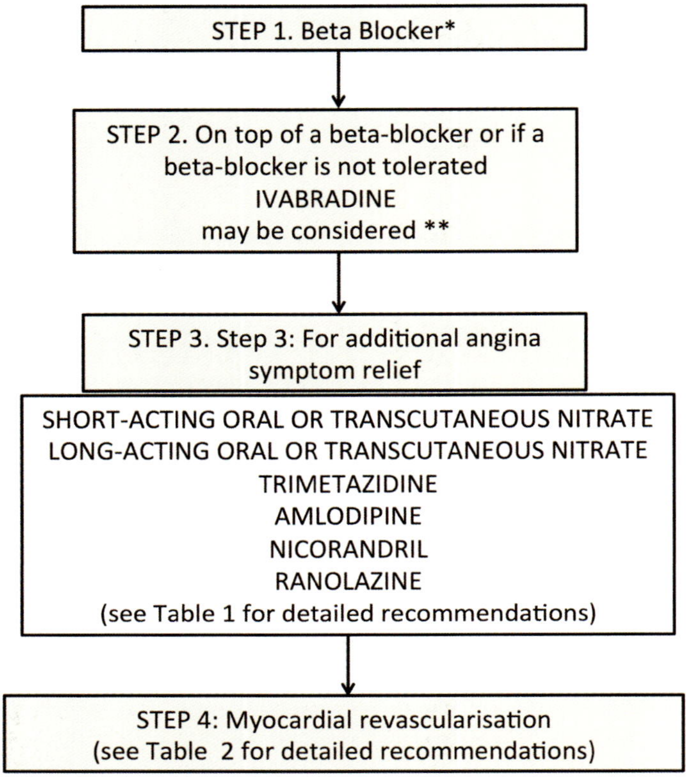

FIGURE 15.1 Treatment of stable angina pectoris patients with symptomatic HFrEF according to 2016 ESC guidelines[1]

*A beta-blocker (in an evidence-based or maximum tolerated dose) is recommended as the preferred first-line treatment to relieve angina because of the associated benefits of this treatment (reducing the risk of HF hospitalization and the risk of premature death).

**Ivabradine should be considered as an anti-anginal drug in suitable HFrEF patients (sinus rhythm and heart rate $\geq$ 70 bpm) as per recommended HFrEF management.

bpm = beats per minute; HF = heart failure; HFrEF = heart failure with reduced ejection fraction

improve New York Heart Association functional class, exercise duration and left ventricular function[9–15] and therefore according to the guidelines[1] trimetazidine may be beneficial and safe in patients with HFrEF for added angina control.

Anti-anginal drugs such as amlodipine.[15] nicorandil[16] and nitrates[17,18] have all been found to be safe and efficacious symptom-wise in HFrEF patients

TABLE 15.1 ESC recommendations for additional angina symptom relief* in patients with symptomatic HFrEF

Recommendation	Class
A short-acting oral or transcutaneous nitrate should be considered (effective anti-anginal treatment, safe in HF).	IIa
A long acting oral or transcutaneous nitrate should be considered (effective anti-anginal treatment, not extensively studied in HF).	IIa
Trimetazidine may be considered when angina persists despite treatment with a beta-blocker (or alternative) to relieve angina (effective anti-anginal treatment, safe in HF).	IIb
Amlodipine may be considered in patients unable to tolerate a beta-blocker to relieve angina (effective anti-anginal treatment, safe in HF).	IIb
Nicorandil may be considered in patients unable to tolerate a beta-blocker to relieve angina (effective anti-anginal treatment, but safety in HF uncertain).	IIb
Ranolazine may be considered in patients unable to tolerate a beta-blocker to relieve angina (effective anti-anginal treatment, but safety in HF uncertain).	IIb

* except from any combination not recommended

HF = heart failure; HFrEF = Heart failure with reduced ejection fraction.

Class of recommendation: I = evidence and/or general agreement that a given treatment or procedure is beneficial, useful, effective; II = conflicting evidence and/or a divergence of opinion about the usefulness/efficacy of the given treatment or procedure (IIa: weight of evidence/opinion is in favor of usefulness/efficacy; IIb: usefulness/efficacy is less well established by evidence/opinion); III: evidence or general agreement that the given treatment or procedure is not useful/effective, and in some cases may be harmful.

with angina. On the contrary, there is evidence that diltiazem and verapamil are unsafe in HFrEF, although they may be used in HFpEF patients.[19] Finally, the safety of ranolazine and dihydropyridine CCBs (except amlodipine[15] and felodipine[20]) remains to be clarified.

Percutaneous and surgical revascularisation

Relief of angina symptoms in HFpEF may be obtained by myocardial revascularisation.[1] Unfortunately, it still remains to be clarified whether revascularisation procedures would also improve the prognosis. According to the ESC guidelines on myocardial revascularisation[21] and to the ESC guidelines on stable CAD,[22] coronary artery bypass grafting (CABG) is recommended to improve prognosis for patients with significant left main stenosis and/or proximal stenosis of both left anterior descending and left circumflex arteries (left main equivalent). However, further studies are needed to substantiate and

TABLE 15.2 ESC recommendations for myocardial revascularisation in patients with stable angina and symptomatic HFrEF

Recommendation	Class
Myocardial revascularization is recommended when angina persists despite treatment with anti-anginal drugs.	I
Alternatives to myocardial revascularization: combination of > 3 anti-anginal drugs (from those listed above) may be considered when angina persists despite treatment with a beta-blocker, ivabradine and an extra anti-anginal drug (excluding the combinations not recommended below).	IIb
The following are NOT recommended: 1. Combination of any of ivabradine, ranolazine, and nicorandil because of unknown safety 2. Combination of nicorandil and a nitrate (because of lack of additional efficacy)	III
Diltiazem and verapamil are not recommended because of their negative inotropic action and risk of worsening HF.	III

HF = heart failure; HFrEF = Heart failure with reduced ejection fraction

Class of recommendation: I = evidence and/or general agreement that a given treatment or procedure is beneficial, useful, effective; II = conflicting evidence and/or a divergence of opinion about the usefulness/efficacy of the given treatment or procedure (IIa: weight of evidence/opinion is in favor of usefulness/efficacy; IIb: usefulness/efficacy is less well established by evidence/opinion); III: evidence or general agreement that the given treatment or procedure is not useful/effective, and in some cases may be harmful.

extend this recommendation to patient with an established diagnosis of HF who formed a very small part of these mainly historical studies upon which this recommendation has been based. The Surgical Treatment for Ischemic Heart Failure (STICH) trial[23] demonstrated the efficacy and safety of CABG in patients with HFrEF and significant CAD (left anterior descending artery or multivessel disease) to reduce death and hospitalisation for cardiovascular causes. In particular, those with >10% of dysfunctional but viable LV myocardium were more likely to benefit from myocardial revascularisation (and those with ≤ 10% less likely to benefit), although further studies are needed to support these conclusions.[1]

According to the 2016 ESC/HFA guidelines, the clinician should make the decision between CABG and percutaneous coronary intervention (PCI) after the careful assessment of patient's clinical status including the prevalent coronary anatomy and site of stenoses, the expected completeness of revascularisation, and any coexisting valvular disease or other co-morbidities.

References

1. Ponikowski P, Voors AA, Anker SD, Bueno H, Cleland JG, Coats AJ, et al. The Task Force for the diagnosis and treatment of acute and chronic heart failure of the European Society of Cardiology (ESC) Developed with the special contribution of the Heart Failure Association (HFA) of the ESC. Eur Heart J. 2016 May 20. pii: ehw128. PMID: 27206819.
2. Braunstein, J. B., G. F. Anderson, G. Gerstenblith, W. Weller, M. Niefeld, R. Herbert and A. W. Wu (2003). Noncardiac comorbidity increases preventable hospitalizations and mortality among Medicare beneficiaries with chronic heart failure. J Am Coll Cardiol 42(7): 1226–1233.
3. Jolicoeur, E. M., A. Dunning, S. Castelvecchio, R. Dabrowski, M. A. Waclawiw, M. C. Petrie, R. Stewart, P. S. Jhund, P. Desvigne-Nickens, J. A. Panza, R. O. Bonow, B. Sun, T. R. San, H. R. Al-Khalidi, J. L. Rouleau, E. J. Velazquez and J. G. Cleland (2015). Importance of angina in patients with coronary disease, heart failure, and left ventricular systolic dysfunction: insights from STICH. J Am Coll Cardiol 66(19): 2092–2100.
4. Flather, M. D., M. C. Shibata, A. J. Coats, D. J. Van Veldhuisen, A. Parkhomenko, J. Borbola, A. Cohen-Solal, D. Dumitrascu, R. Ferrari, P. Lechat, J. Soler-Soler, L. Tavazzi, L. Spinarova, J. Toman, M. Bohm, S. D. Anker, S. G. Thompson, P. A. Poole-Wilson and S. Investigators (2005). Randomized trial to determine the effect of nebivolol on mortality and cardiovascular hospital admission in elderly patients with heart failure (SENIORS). Eur Heart J 26(3): 215–225.
5. Fonarow, G. C., W. G. Stough, W. T. Abraham, N. M. Albert, M. Gheorghiade, B. H. Greenberg, C. M. O'Connor, J. L. Sun, C. W. Yancy, J. B. Young, O.-H. Investigators and Hospitals (2007). Characteristics, treatments, and outcomes of patients with preserved systolic function hospitalized for heart failure: a report from the OPTIMIZE-HF Registry. J Am Coll Cardiol 50(8): 768–777.
6. Ambrosio, G., M. D. Flather, M. Bohm, A. Cohen-Solal, A. Murrone, F. Mascagni, G. Spinucci, M. G. Conti, D. J. van Veldhuisen, L. Tavazzi and A. J. Coats (2011). beta-blockade with nebivolol for prevention of acute ischaemic events in elderly patients with heart failure. Heart 97(3): 209–214.
7. Bohm, M., A. Link, D. Cai, M. S. Nieminen, G. S. Filippatos, R. Salem, A. Cohen Solal, B. Huang, R. J. Padley, M. Kivikko and A. Mebazaa (2011). Beneficial association of beta-blocker therapy on recovery from severe acute heart failure treatment: data from the Survival of Patients With Acute Heart Failure in Need of Intravenous Inotropic Support trial. Crit Care Med 39(5): 940–944.
8. Swedberg, K., M. Komajda, M. Bohm, J. S. Borer, I. Ford, A. Dubost-Brama, G. Lerebours, L. Tavazzi and S. Investigators (2010). Ivabradine and outcomes in chronic heart failure (SHIFT): a randomised placebo-controlled study. Lancet 376(9744): 875–885.
9. Rosano, G. M., C. Vitale, B. Sposato, G. Mercuro and M. Fini (2003). Trimetazidine improves left ventricular function in diabetic patients with coronary artery disease: a double-blind placebo-controlled study. Cardiovasc Diabetol 2: 16.
10. Vitale, C., M. Wajngaten, B. Sposato, O. Gebara, P. Rossini, M. Fini, M. Volterrani and

G. M. Rosano (2004). Trimetazidine improves left ventricular function and quality of life in elderly patients with coronary artery disease. Eur Heart J 25(20): 1814–1821.

11. Marazzi, G., M. Wajngarten, C. Vitale, R. Patrizi, F. Pelliccia, O. Gebara, H. Pierri, J. A. Ramires, M. Volterrani, M. Fini and G. M. Rosano (2007). Effect of free fatty acid inhibition on silent and symptomatic myocardial ischemia in diabetic patients with coronary artery disease. Int J Cardiol 120(1): 79–84.
12. Marazzi, G., O. Gebara, C. Vitale, G. Caminiti, M. Wajngarten, M. Volterrani, J. A. Ramires, G. Rosano and M. Fini (2009). Effect of trimetazidine on quality of life in elderly patients with ischemic dilated cardiomyopathy. Adv Ther 26(4): 455–461.
13. Gao, D., N. Ning, X. Niu, G. Hao and Z. Meng (2011). Trimetazidine: a meta-analysis of randomised controlled trials in heart failure. Heart 97(4): 278–286.
14. Vitale, C., I. Spoletini, W. Malorni, P. Perrone-Filardi, M. Volterrani and G. M. Rosano (2013). Efficacy of trimetazidine on functional capacity in symptomatic patients with stable exertional angina – the VASCO-angina study. Int J Cardiol 168(2): 1078–1081.
15. Packer, M., C. M. O'Connor, J. K. Ghali, M. L. Pressler, P. E. Carson, R. N. Belkin, A. B. Miller, G. W. Neuberg, D. Frid, J. H. Wertheimer, A. B. Cropp and D. L. DeMets (1996). Effect of amlodipine on morbidity and mortality in severe chronic heart failure. Prospective Randomized Amlodipine Survival Evaluation Study Group. N Engl J Med 335(15): 1107–1114.
16. (Iona Study Group 2002). Effect of nicorandil on coronary events in patients with stable angina: the Impact Of Nicorandil in Angina (IONA) randomised trial. Lancet 359(9314): 1269–1275.
17. Cohn, J. N., D. G. Archibald, S. Ziesche, J. A. Franciosa, W. E. Harston, F. E. Tristani, W. B. Dunkman, W. Jacobs, G. S. Francis, K. H. Flohr and et al. (1986). Effect of vasodilator therapy on mortality in chronic congestive heart failure. Results of a Veterans Administration Cooperative Study. N Engl J Med 314(24): 1547–1552.
18. Cohn, J. N., G. Johnson, S. Ziesche, F. Cobb, G. Francis, F. Tristani, R. Smith, W. B. Dunkman, H. Loeb, M. Wong and et al. (1991). A comparison of enalapril with hydralazine-isosorbide dinitrate in the treatment of chronic congestive heart failure. N Engl J Med 325(5): 303–310.
19. Goldstein, R. E., S. J. Boccuzzi, D. Cruess and S. Nattel (1991). Diltiazem increases late-onset congestive heart failure in postinfarction patients with early reduction in ejection fraction. The Adverse Experience Committee; and the Multicenter Diltiazem Postinfarction Research Group. Circulation 83(1): 52–60.
20. Cohn, J. N., S. Ziesche, R. Smith, I. Anand, W. B. Dunkman, H. Loeb, G. Cintron, W. Boden, L. Baruch, P. Rochin and L. Loss (1997). Effect of the calcium antagonist felodipine as supplementary vasodilator therapy in patients with chronic heart failure treated with enalapril: V-HeFT III. Vasodilator-Heart Failure Trial (V-HeFT) Study Group. Circulation 96(3): 856–863.
21. Windecker, S., P. Kolh, F. Alfonso, J. P. Collet, J. Cremer, V. Falk, G. Filippatos, C. Hamm, S. J. Head, P. Juni, A. P. Kappetein, A. Kastrati, J. Knuuti, U. Landmesser, G. Laufer, F. J. Neumann, D. J. Richter, P. Schauerte, M. Sousa Uva, G. G. Stefanini, D. P. Taggart, L. Torracca, M. Valgimigli, W. Wijns and A. Witkowski (2015). 2014 ESC/EACTS guidelines on myocardial revascularization. EuroIntervention 10(9): 1024–1094.

22. Montalescot, G., U. Sechtem, S. Achenbach, F. et al. (2013). 2013 ESC guidelines on the management of stable coronary artery disease: the Task Force on the management of stable coronary artery disease of the European Society of Cardiology. Eur Heart J 34(38): 2949–3003.
23. Velazquez, E. J., K. L. Lee, M. A. Deja, A. Jain, G. Sopko, A. Marchenko, I. S. Ali, G. Pohost, S. Gradinac, W. T. Abraham, M. Yii, D. Prabhakaran, H. Szwed, P. Ferrazzi, M. C. Petrie, C. M. O'Connor, P. Panchavinnin, L. She, R. O. Bonow, G. R. Rankin, R. H. Jones, J. L. Rouleau and S. Investigators (2011). Coronary-artery bypass surgery in patients with left ventricular dysfunction. N Engl J Med. 364(17): 1607–1616.

16

The management of co-morbidities in patients with heart failure – hypertension

Background

The 2016 ESC/HFA HF guidelines carry an important section on the treatments of co-morbidities in HF.[1] Foremost of these in terms of frequency and its relevance to the aetiology of HF, especially HFpEF is hypertension. In this chapter we will review what the recent guidelines say about the management of hypertension in the setting of HF, both HFrEF and HFpEF and expand on some of the practical advice.

These guidelines carry an extremely important guidance table (reproduced in Figure 16.1). This table carries an enormous amount of important advice, for it outlines the progressive steps in using evidence-based medicines to manage the hypertensive HF patient, in which order to try agents and how to progressively increase the drug treatment armamentarium used. It also summarises in a colour and alphanumeric schema the strength of the recommendation and the strength of the underlying evidence, and then in addition it importantly points out those otherwise widely used agents which should NOT be used in the setting of HF where they would form part of any conventional hypertension guidelines for patients not having co-morbid heart failure. It therefore deserves a much closer look.

In the preamble to this guidance table it is pointed out that hypertension is a potent risk factor for HF (and for HFpEF even more than for HFrEF); that antihypertensive therapy markedly reduces the incidence of HF and that although good control of high blood pressure is essential in all HF patients,

Recommendations	Class [a]	Level [b]
Step 1		
ACE-I (or ARB), a beta-blocker or an MRA (or a combination) is recommended to reduce blood pressure as first-, second- and third-line therapy, respectively, because of their associated benefits in HFrEF (reducing the risk of death and HF hospitalization). They are also safe in HFpEF.	I	A
Step 2		
A thiazide diuretic (or if the patient is being treated with a thiazide diuretic, switching to a loop diuretic) is recommended to reduce blood pressure when hypertension persists despite treatment with a combination of an ACE-I (or alternatively ARB but NOT together withan ACE-I), a beta-blocker and an MRA.	I	C
Step 3		
Amlodipine or hydralazine is recommended to reduce blood pressure when hypertension persists despite treatment with a combination of an ACE-I (or alternatively ARB but NOT together withan ACE-I), a beta-blocker, an MRA and a diuretic.	I	A
Felodipine should be considered to reduce blood pressure when hypertension persists despite treatment with a combination of an ACE-I (or alternatively ARB but NOT together withan ACE-I), a beta-blocker, an MRA and a diuretic.	IIa	B
Moxonidine is not recommended to reduce blood pressure because of safety concerns in HFrEF patients (increased mortality).	III	B
Alpha-adrenoceptor antagonists are not recommended to reduce blood pressure because of safety concerns in HFrEF patients (neurohormonal activation, fluid retention, worsening HF).	III	A
Diltiazem and verapamil are not recommended to reduce blood pressure in patients with HFrEF because of their negative inotropic action and risk of worsening HF.	III	C

FIGURE 16.1 The 2016 ESC/HFA guidelines[1] guidance for the management of hypertension complicating heart failure.

poor control in advanced HFrEF is actually extremely uncommon, whereas it is a much more important problem in milder HFrEF cases and in HFmrEF and HFpEF in particular. HF has not been a prominent end-point in many hypertension trials. Despite this there is a consistent and powerful protection from HF that can be achieved by treating hypertension that appears related to the BP control rather than the choice of agent, with the sole exception that alpha-adrenoceptor blockers appear less effective than other drug classes in this effect.[2] Good BP control is an essential part of the management of the HF patients with prospective observations showing in HF patients followed long term, higher baseline systolic, diastolic and pulse pressure levels were associated with higher rates of adverse events.[3] BP targets are the same as in the non-HF hypertensive patient (<140/90 by repeated office BP measurement in most, between 140–150 in elderly with starting SBP's >160 mmHg) with a lower DBP target for diabetics (<85 mmHg).[4] The value of more intensive BP control in hypertensive HF patients remains to be clarified.

The steps to good BP control in heart failure

Step 1 in any hypertensive HF patient is to use an ACE inhibitor (or ARB only if such is not tolerated), a beta blocker and an MRA. As anyone with significant HF will already be recommended a beta blocker an ACEI and a MRA there is really little of clinical change to make here, the main difference being the prominent position of beta-blockade as opposed to this drug class's relative demotion in non-HF hypertension guidelines. Step 2, should greater BP control be needed after the drugs is step one have all been started and up-titrated is to commence a thiazide diuretic (or if the patient is treated with a thiazide diuretic, switching to a loop diuretic). Care will need to be taken if already on loop diuretics for HF as combination diuretics can cause severe fluid depletion, renal impairment and electrolyte disturbances. Step 3 (which will rarely be needed in moderate to severe HFrEF) is to add a calcium channel blocker, but here the choice of agent is critical. Amlodipine and to a lesser extent Felodipine have been shown to be safe in HFrEF.[5,6] If an alternative is needed hydralazine can be added (but should not be used without the ACEi and beta blockers of the earlier steps).[7]

Importantly advice is given in which drugs should never be used in the setting of HF (despite being in hypertension guidelines). These include Moxonidine, alpha receptor antagonists, diltiazem and verapamil, although the latter two are probably safe in HFpEF, because the concern in HFrEF is their negative inotropic effect which is of less concern in true HFpEF. Moxonidine increased mortality in patients in the MOXCON trial in HFrEF[8] and there are concerns of the risk in HFrEF patients of neurohormonal activation, fluid retention and worsening HF with alpha-adrenoceptor antagonists.[9–11]

Lastly in the setting of acute heart failure (AHF) i.v. nitrates (or sodium nitroprusside, starting with 0.3 μg/kg/min and increasing up to 5 μg/kg/min) are recommended to lower blood pressure. For AHF with uncontrolled hypertension (mostly HFpEF rather than HFrEF) Isosorbide dinitrate infusion is recommended starting with 1 mg/h, increasing up to 10 mg/h.

References

1. Ponikowski P, Voors A, Anker S et al The Task Force for the diagnosis and treatment of acute and chronic heart failure of the European Society of Cardiology (ESC). 2016 ESC Guidelines for the diagnosis and treatment of acute and chronic heart failure. European Journal of Heart Failure. Published online 26 May 2016.
2. Major cardiovascular events in hypertensive patients randomized to doxazosin vs chlorthalidone. ALLHAT Collaborative Research Group. JAMA 2000; 283: 1967–1975.
3. Lip GYH, Skjøth F, Overvad K, Rasmussen LH, Larsen TB. Blood pressure and prognosis in patients with incident heart failure: the Diet, Cancer and Health (DCH) cohort study. Clin Res Cardiol 2015; 104: 1088–1096.
4. Giuseppe Mancia, Robert Fagard, Krzysztof Narkiewicz, et al. 2013 ESH/ESC Guidelines for the management of arterial hypertension European Heart Journal 2013; 34: 2159–2219. doi:http://dx.doi.org/10.1093/eurheartj/eht151
5. Packer M, O'Connor CM, Ghali JK, Pressler ML, Carson PE, Belkin RN, Miller AB, Neuberg GW, Frid D, Wertheimer JH, Cropp AB, DeMets DL. Effect of amlodipine on morbidity and mortality in severe chronic heart failure. Prospective Randomized Amlodipine Survival Evaluation Study Group. N Engl J Med 1996; 335: 1107–1114.
6. Cohn JN, Ziesche S, Smith R, Anand I, Dunkman WB, Loeb H, Cintron G, Boden W,

Baruch L, Rochin P, Loss L. Effect of the calcium antagonist felodipine as supplementary vasodilator therapy in patients with chronic heart failure treated with enalapril: V-HeFT III. Vasodilator-Heart Failure Trial (V-HeFT) Study Group. Circulation 1997; 96: 856–863.

7. Taylor AL, Ziesche S, Yancy C, Carson P, D'Agostino R, Ferdinand K, Taylor M, Adams K, Sabolinski M, Worcel M, Cohn JN. Combination of isosorbide dinitrate and hydralazine in blacks with heart failure. N Engl J Med 2004; 351: 2049–2057.
8. Cohn JN, Pfeffer MA, Rouleau J, Sharpe N, Swedberg K, Straub M, Wiltse C, Wright TJ, MOXCON Investigators. Adverse mortality effect of central sympathetic inhibition with sustained-release moxonidine in patients with heart failure (MOXCON). Eur J Heart Fail 2003; 5: 659–667.
9. The ALLHAT Officers and Coordinators for the ALLHAT Collaborative Research Group. Major Cardiovascular Events in Hypertensive Patients Randomized to Doxazosin vs Chlorthalidone. JAMA J Am Med Assoc 2000; 283: 1967–1975.
10. Dorszewski A, Göhmann E, Dorszewski B, Werner GS, Kreuzer H, Figulla HR. Vasodilation by urapidil in the treatment of chronic congestive heart failure in addition to angiotensin-converting enzyme inhibitors is not beneficial: results of a placebo-controlled, double-blind study. J Card Fail 1997; 3: 91–96.
11. Bayliss J, Norell MS, Canepa-Anson R, Reid C, Poole-Wilson P, Sutton G. Clinical importance of the renin-angiotensin system in chronic heart failure: double blind comparison of captopril and prazosin. Br Med J (Clin Res Ed) 1985; 290: 1861–1865.

17

Valvular heart disease in heart failure

Structural valvular heart disease may be the cause of heart failure or may worsen the clinical status of patients with heart failure. Heart failure may also develop in patients treated with valve surgery.[1,2] Patients with heart failure with valvular heart disease are at increased risk of events including sudden cardiac death. Before considering intervention (surgical or percutaneous) all patients should receive appropriate medical and device therapy taking into account that vasodilators must be used with caution in patients with severe aortic stenosis. Numerous percutaneous and/or hybrid procedures have been introduced in the past few years and they are changing the management of valvular heart disease.

Aortic stenosis

Aortic stenosis occurs in nearly 2.8% of patients ≥75 years of age and can occur because of degenerative calcification and congenital valvular defects such as bicuspid aortic valves or as one of the sequelae of rheumatic disease.[3]

One of the major tasks in patients with HFrEf with aortic valve disease is the adequate assessment of the degree of stenosis since 'low-flow, low-gradient' aortic stenosis (ΔPmean <40 mm Hg) can be both a pseudostenosis due to a co-existent cardiomyopathy or be a manifestation of a significant underestimation of the degree of aortic stenosis and its clinical significance because of the added effects of diseased left ventricle reducing the pressure head driving blood across the diseased valve.[4] Patients with pseudostenosis have moderately diseased aortic valves with impaired leaflet opening because of the reduced left ventricular function. The identification of pseudostenosis is of crucial importance since, unlike true aortic stenosis, it carries a high mortality risk (nearly 50%) with surgical aortic valve replacement while it benefits more from medical therapy for heart failure.[5] Dobutamine stress either during echocardiography or catheterization is the main method of differentiating pseudostenosis from true aortic valve stenosis. During the dobutamine test the contractility increases the stroke volume and will increase the trans-aortic pressure gradient and velocity while the effective orifice area will not change in the patient with true severe aortic stenosis. In patients with pseudostenosis, dobutamine infusion with the consequent increase in stroke volume will open the aortic valve causing no change in pressure gradient and velocity resulting in an increased calculated valve area confirming the moderate degree of aortic stenosis.[4,5]

In symptomatic patients with heart failure and a mean gradient >40 mmHg, left ventricular function is not a limitation for aortic valve replacement. In patients with heart failure and severe aortic stenosis who are not suitable for surgery as assessed by a 'heart team' Transaortic valve implantation (TAVI) is recommended if a post-TAVI survival of at least one year is predicted. The heart team has a central role in deciding whether TAVI should be also considered in high-risk patients with heart failure and severe aortic stenosis who may be suitable for surgery, but in whom TAVI is favoured on the basis of individual risk profile and anatomic appropriateness.[6–9] The field of TAVI is quickly evolving and recent trials in patients with both moderate and severe aortic stenosis have shown that TAVI confers a significantly higher rate of event free survival at 1 year.[6–9]

Aortic regurgitation

Aortic regurgitation (AR) increases the load on the left ventricular in ventricles with already reduced function and therefore significantly aggravates heart failure. Aortic valve repair or replacement is recommended in all patients with heart failure who are symptomatic and have severe aortic regurgitation and in those who are asymptomatic with severe AR but otherwise fit for surgery.[10,11]

Mitral regurgitation

Patients with heart failure may present with mitral regurgitation (MR) because of a primary valve disease or rupture or may represent a functional consequence of a dilated hypokinetic left ventricle.

In symptomatic patients with severe organic MR with no contra-indications mitral valve replacement is indicated.[12–13] Available surgical expertise is a major factor in deciding whether to replace or repair the mitral valve but the decision is individualised by the heart team and depends on factors such as mitral valve anatomy, co-existing coronary disease, other co-morbidities and the overall clinical condition of the patient.

Although surgical repair may durably improve symptoms, its long term effect on survival in patients with HFrEF and left ventricular EF <30% is unknown. In this condition, the decision to operate should take into account the overall clinical status, the presence of co-morbidities and the response to medical therapy. In this case the choice to repair or replace the mitral valve lies with the surgical team.[12–13]

Functional mitral regurgitation

Functional mitral regurgitation (FMR) is the consequence of left ventricular enlargement and remodelling that leads to reduced mitral valve leaflet closure and coaptation. FMR is often present in patients with HFrEF and is a marker of adverse outcomes and poor long-term survival when present.[14,15] FMR may be variable and can also contribute to progressive left ventricular dilatation and dysfunction and worsened symptoms. Anatomical changes can lead to a progression of FMR with an average annual increase of 5– 8 ml in regurgitant volume and 4–6 mm^2 in the effective regurgitant orifice area.[16]

In patients with FMR, the valvular apparatus (papillary muscles, chordae, and valve leaflets) is typically normal. Mitral leaflet mal-coaptation and mitral valve regurgitation may result from a combination of papillary muscle displacement due to left ventricular remodeling, decreased systolic closing force and annular enlargement secondary to left ventricular dilatation. Progression of left ventricular dilation and remodeling, aggravated by the volume overload imposed by FMR, amplifies leaflet tethering increasing the inter-papillary muscle distance and a lateral redirection of the tethering forces, which are normally perpendicular to the mitral annular plane, resulting in a furher progression of FMR.[17]

Effective medical therapy (including CRT in patients with clear indications) may reverse left ventricular remodelling and may reduce FMR. Therefore, every effort should be made first to optimize medical treatment in patients with heart failure presenting with FMR. In symptomatic patients with heart failure of ischaemic origin and left ventricular EF <30% combined valve and coronary surgery should be considered if there is evidence of myocardial viability and a coronary anatomy suitable for revascularization. Mitral valve surgery is recommended also in those patients with heart failure and left ventricular function <30% and severe mitral regurgitation undergoing CABG.[18] The addition of mitral valve repair to CABG, however, has not clearly proven to have a significant effect on left ventricular reverse remodeling in patients with moderate, secondary ischaemic mitral regurgitation as there is no evidence favouring mitral valve repair over replacement. In patients with heart failure and FMR and atrial fibrillation, atrial ablation and LA appendage closure may be considered at the time of mitral valve surgery.

In patients with severe FMR and severe left ventricular dysfunction (LVEF <30%) who have non-ischaemic cardiomyopathy or who are not suitable for myocardial revascularisation the indication for mitral valve surgery is debatable, and medical and device therapy is to be preferred, even though in selected patients mitral valve repair may be considered in order to slow the progression of the disease.[18] In patients with heart failure and moderate-severe FMR who are judged at high surgical risk, percutaneous edge-to-edge repair with the Mitra-Clip device or with newer devices may be considered in order to improve symptoms and quality of life. However there is no evidence that this approach leads to any long term prognostic improvement.[19,20]

Tricuspid regurgitation

Primary tricuspid regurgitation (TR) is an extremely rare cause of heart failure. In secondary tricuspid regurgitation the leaflets and chords themselves are not primarily affected but the tricuspid annulus stretches because of right ventricular failure or enlargement as a consequence of elevated pulmonary pressures. Functional tricuspid regurgitation frequently complicates the natural course of patients with heart failure. A "V" wave on the jugular venous pulse is a clear sign of tricuspid regurgitation in patients with heart failure. When tricuspid regurgitation becomes severe it may worsen symptoms of right heart failure.

In these patients adequate diuretic therapy is important also because hepatic congestion that is often present in these patients may contribute to hyperaldosteronism. Therefore, the addition of an MRA (at higher natriuretic doses) may improve decongestion.[21] There are presently no clear indications for surgical correction of functional TR in patients with heart failure.[18] The correction of TR, if appropriate, may be considered at the time of surgical correction of left-sided valve lesions but this is a decision to be taken on an individual patient level taking into account the fact that the additonal procedure prolongs surgical procedure times and therefore risk. Although catheter-based interventions have been proposed for the correction of functional tricuspid regurgitation, their role and safety remains inadequately studied.[22]

Conclusions

In patients with heart failure and valvular heart disease, either primary or functional, the whole process of decision-making should be staged through a comprehensive evaluation of the risk– benefit ratio of different treatment strategies and should be made by a multidisciplinary 'heart team' with a particular expertise in valvular heart disease. The heart team should include heart failure cardiologists, cardiac surgeons/structural valve interventionists, imaging specialists, anaesthetists, geriatricians and intensive care specialists.

References

1. Vahanian A, Alfieri O, Andreotti F, et al. Guidelines on the management of valvular heart disease (version 2012): the Joint Task Force on the Management of Valvular Heart Disease of the European Society of Cardiology (ESC) and the European Association for Cardio-Thoracic Surgery (EACTS). Eur Heart J 2012; 33: 2451–2496.
2. Nishimura RA, Otto CM, Bonow RO, et al. 2014 AHA/ACC guideline for the management of patients with valvular heart disease: executive summary: a report of the American College of Cardiology/American Heart Association Task Force on Practice Guidelines. J Am Coll Cardiol 2014; 63: 2438–2488.
3. Carabello BA, Paulus WJ. Aortic stenosis. Lancet. 2009; 373: 956–966.
4. Clark C. Relation between pressure difference across the aortic valve and left ventricular outflow. Cardiovasc Res. 1978; 12: 276–287.
5. Dumesnil JG, Pibarot P, Carabello B. Paradoxical low flow and/or low gradient severe aortic stenosis despite preserved left ventricular ejection fraction: implications for diagnosis and treatment. Eur Heart J. 2010; 31: 281–289.
6. Smith CR, Leon MB, Mack MJ, et al. Transcatheter versus surgical aortic-valve replacement in high-risk patients. N Engl J Med 2011; 364: 2187–2198.
7. Leon MB, Smith CR, Mack M, et al. Transcatheter aortic-valve implantation for aortic stenosis in patients who cannot undergo surgery. N Engl J Med 2010; 363: 1597–1607.
8. Reardon MJ, Adams DH, Kleiman NS, et al. 2-Year outcomes in patients undergoing surgical or self-expanding transcatheter aortic valve replacement. J Am Coll Cardiol 2015; 66: 113–121.
9. Adams DH, Popma JJ, Reardon MJ, et al. Transcatheter aortic-valve replacement with a self-expanding prosthesis. N Engl J Med 2014; 370: 1790–1798.
10. Lancellotti P, Tribouilloy C, Hagendorff A, et al. Recommendations for the echocardiographic assessment of native valvular regurgitation: an executive summary from the European Association of Cardiovascular Imaging. Eur Heart J Cardiovasc Imaging 2013; 14: 611–644.
11. Chaliki HP, Mohty D, Avierinos JF, et al. Outcomes after aortic valve replacement in patients with severe aortic regurgitation and markedly reduced left ventricular function. Circulation 2002; 106: 2687–2693.
12. Smith PK, Puskas JD, Ascheim DD, et al. Surgical treatment of moderate ischemic mitral regurgitation. N Engl J Med 2014; 371: 2178–2188.

13. Acker MA, Parides MK, Perrault LP, et al. Mitral-valve repair versus replacement for severe ischemic mitral regurgitation. N Engl J Med 2014; 370: 23–32.
14. Lebrun F, Patrizi P, Pierard L. Quantitation of functional mitral regurgitation during bicycle exercise in patients with heart failure. Journal of the American College of Cardiology 2001: 38: 1685–1692.
15. Schmitto JD, Lee LS, et al. Functional mitral regurgitation Cardiology Review 2010 Nov – Dec; 18(6): 285–91.
16. Michelena H, Valentina B, et al. Progress in the Treatment of Severe Mitral Regurgitation – Rev Esp Cardiology 2010; 63: 820–31 – Vol. 63 Num 07.
17. Otsuji Y, Handschumacher MD, Schwammenthal E, et al. Insights from three-dimensional echocardiography into the mechanism of functional mitral regurgitation: direct in vivo demonstration of altered leaflet tethering geometry. Circulation 1997; 96: 1999–2008.
18. Ponikowski P, Voors AA, Anker SD, Bueno H, Cleland JG, Coats AJ, Falk V, González-Juanatey JR, Harjola VP, Jankowska EA, Jessup M, Linde C, Nihoyannopoulos P, Parissis JT, Pieske B, Riley JP, Rosano GM, Ruilope LM, Ruschitzka F, Rutten FH, van der Meer P. 2016 ESC Guidelines for the diagnosis and treatment of acute and chronic heart failure: The Task Force for the diagnosis and treatment of acute and chronic heart failure of the European Society of Cardiology (ESC). Developed with the special contribution of the Heart Failure Association (HFA) of the ESC. Eur J Heart Fail. 2016 May 20.
19. D'ascenzo F, Moretti C, Marra WG, et al. Meta-analysis of the usefulness of mitraclip in patients with functional mitral regurgitation. Am J Cardiol 2015; 116: 325–331.
20. Nickenig G, Estevez-Loureiro R, Franzen O, et al. Transcatheter Valve Treatment Sentinel Registry Investigators of the EURObservational Research Programme of the European Society of Cardiology. Percutaneous mitral valve edge-to-edge repair: in-hospital results and 1-year follow-up of 628 patients of the 2011–2012 pilot European Sentinel Registry. J Am Coll Cardiol 2014; 64: 875–884.
21. Perez-Ayuso RM, Arroyo V, Planas R, et al. Randomized comparative study of efficacy of furosemide versus spironolactone in nonazotemic cirrhosis with ascites. Relationship between the diuretic response and the activity of the renin-aldosterone system. Gastroenterology 1983; 84: 961–968.
22. Schofer J, Bijuklic K, Tiburtius C, Hansen L, Groothuis A, Hahn RT. First-in-human transcatheter tricuspid valve repair in a patient with severely regurgitant tricuspid valve. J Am Coll Cardiol 2015; 65: 1190–1195.

18

The management of co-morbidities in patients with heart failure – lung disorders

Background

The 2016 ESC/HFA HF guidelines carry an important section on the treatments of co-morbidities in HF.[1] One of the most common and most confusing, in terms of overlapping symptoms and interfering treatments is the presence of significant lung disorders. In this chapter we will review what the recent guidelines say about the management of lung disorders in the setting of HF, both HFrEF and HFpEF and expand on some of the practical advice. Please note that sleep disordered breathing syndromes are covered in the subsequent two chapters.

The diagnosis of COPD and asthma may be complicated in patients with heart failure. HF itself can cause a non-asthmatic bronchial obstruction that can be variable and which can respond to bronchodilators (because they constrict bronchial vessels and reduce the epithelial wall oedema that is thought to be implicated). The important feature is that this form of reversible airway narrowing is not a contra-indication to beta-blockers which severe classical asthma is. The interpretation of spirometry can be complex especially in HFpEF.[2–4] There are many overlaps between CHF and COPD including vascular remodelling inflammation and cachexia and skeletal muscle wasting. The presence of each increases morbidity and mortality of the other. The cornerstones of therapy are beta-blockers and beta-agonists, which as their modes of action suggest oppose each other's actions. Hospitalizations and associated health care costs are dramatically higher when they co-exist.

To avoid over-diagnosis of COPD and asthma in the setting of CHF spirometry should be performed only in euvolaemic (at least 3 months) patients.[5,6] Whether the COPD diagnosis is accurate or not, it still carries a higher symptom burned and worse prognosis in HFrEF when it is made even clinically without formal testing. Beta-blocker, the mainstay of HFrEF management still offer substantial benefits to such patients, and must therefore be considered only relatively contraindicated in asthma (especially as true life-threatening asthma is extremely rare in most advanced HF patients). Beta-blockers are not contra-indicated in COPD. It is common practice to prescribe a more highly beta-1 selective adrenoceptor antagonist (i.e. bisoprolol, metoprolol succinate, or nebivolol) although no major outcome comparative study has ever been performed. It is, however, a good practical clinical precaution to start with low doses of cardioselective beta-blockers combined with close monitoring for signs of airway obstruction (wheezing, shortness of breath with lengthening of the expiration). These crucial life-saving medicines should be used but only with very close medical supervision in the initiation and up-titration phases.

Lastly it is important to consider the converse, the safety of conventional COPD medication in the setting of HF, especially HFrEF. The long-term safety of cardioactive inhaled pulmonary drugs is uncertain and the need for their use should be reconsidered in patients with HFrEF. Steroids should always be carefully monitored for their effects on blood pressure and congestion and hence worsened HF. Inhaled administration is therefore to be preferred. In the setting of severe AHF one of the recommended therapies, non-invasive ventilation, is safe and effective regardless of the presence of co-incident COPD provided excessive ventilation removing the occasionally crucial carbon dioxide mediated ventilatory is avoided. Such non-invasive ventilation can improve outcomes of patients with acute respiratory failure and acute HF both in the presence or absence of acute pulmonary oedema.

Lastly life-style advice (optimal weight, regular carefully chosen exercise, adherence to medication, supervision by a disease management team and good communications with health care providers) are all similarly beneficial in COPD as they are in CHF, and doubly important for those patients with both.

References

1. Ponikowski P, Voors A, Anker S et al The Task Force for the diagnosis and treatment of acute and chronic heart failure of the European Society of Cardiology (ESC). 2016 ESC Guidelines for the diagnosis and treatment of acute and chronic heart failure. European Journal of Heart Failure. Published online 26 May 2016.
2. Hawkins NM, Virani S, Ceconi C. Heart failure and chronic obstructive pulmonary disease: the challenges facing physicians and health services. Eur Heart J 2013; 34: 2795–2807.
3. Rutten FH, Moons KGM, Cramer M-JM, Grobbee DE, Zuithoff NPA, Lammers J-WJ, Hoes AW. Recognising heart failure in elderly patients with stable chronic obstructive pulmonary disease in primary care: cross sectional diagnostic study. BMJ 2005; 331: 1379.
4. Hawkins NM, Petrie MC, Jhund PS, Chalmers GW, Dunn FG, McMurray JJV. Heart failure and chronic obstructive pulmonary disease: diagnostic pitfalls and epidemiology. Eur J Heart Fail 2009; 11: 130–139.
5. Brenner S, Güder G, Berliner D, Deubner N, Fröhlich K, Ertl G, Jany B, Angermann CE, Störk S. Airway obstruction in systolic heart failure – COPD or congestion? Int J Cardiol 2013; 168: 1910–1916.
6. Güder G, Brenner S, Störk S, Hoes A, Rutten FH. Chronic obstructive pulmonary disease in heart failure: accurate diagnosis and treatment. Eur J Heart Fail 2014; 16: 1–10.

19

The management of co-morbidities in patients with heart failure – obstructive sleep apnoea

Background

Heart failure (HF) patients are older and frequently present with multiple co-morbidities. Co-morbidities worsen patient symptoms and may contribute to the progression of heart failure, increase mortality or limit the therapeutic response to treatment. Obstructive sleep apnoea (OSA) affects 2–4% of the adult population world-wide and is associated with similar risk factors to HF, meaning it is a frequent finding in HF patients, including HFrEF, HFmrEF and HFpEF. OSA has consistently been shown to be associated with hypertension, coronary artery disease, arrhythmias, heart failure, and stroke.[1–2] A thorough understanding of the diagnosis and treatment options of OSA is of paramount importance to the practising HF clinician. Patients may present to the HF specialist having been diagnosed by a formal sleep study or may be suspected of OSA because of symptoms of snoring, reports of obstructed breathing by the sleep partner or day-time sleepiness.

OSA is caused by upper airway obstruction, usually associated with upper airway collapse. OSA manifests as intermittent airway occlusions, accompanied by consequent loss of airflow, arterial deoxygenation and arousal due to the stimulatory effects of chemoreflex firing secondary to the disturbed arterial blood gases. These obstructive apnoeas or hypopnoeas can occur throughout sleep and are somewhat irregular and are quite distinct form another sleep disordered breathing pattern seen in CHF, central sleep apnoea.[3] The

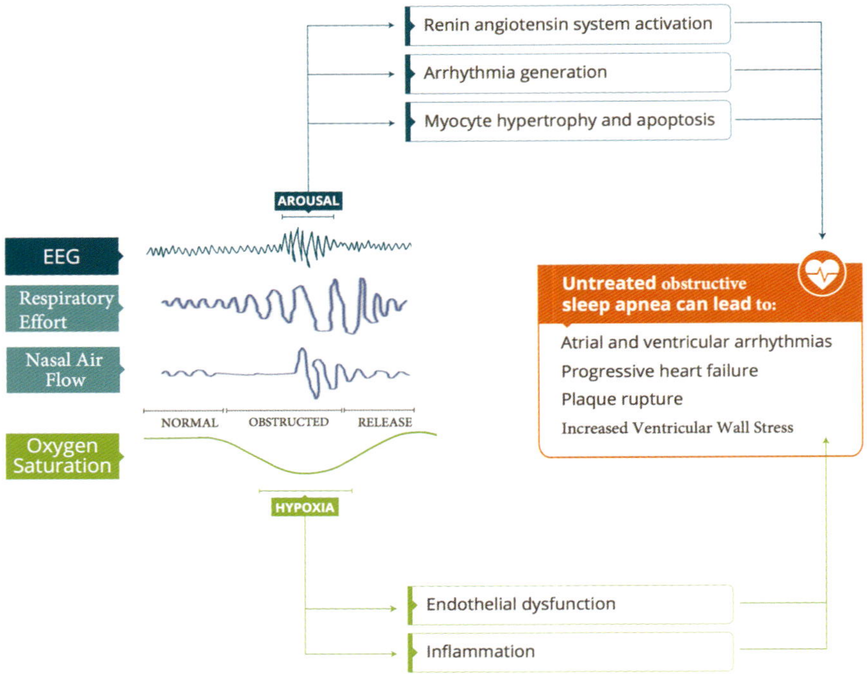

FIGURE 19.1 The pathophysiological consequences of OSA in heart failure

mechanisms underlying the development of OSA in HF are no different to those in patients without HF, but a mixed apnoea pattern is more likely due to respiratory control system instability with subsequent oscillations of the arterial blood carbon dioxide levels ($PaCO_2$) and ventilatory drive due to lung congestion, reduced cardiac output, prolonged circulation times and elevated chemosensitivity.[4–5] Although large-scale trial evidence is lacking physicians are advised to treat HF patients with sleep disordered breathing as OSA if the hypoxias are predominantly obstructive in nature and as CSA (see central sleep apnoea chapter) if the hypoxias are predominantly central in nature.

Pathophysiology

Each OSA cycle of apnoea or hyperpnoea is to an extent independent. The initiating factor is usually airway collapse causing an obstruction to airflow and consequent loss of effective breathing. Hypoxia and consequent arousal (and a surge in sympathetic activity) increases sufficiently to awaken the patient enough such that the airway is opened and effective breathing can resume. Frequent episodes of airway obstruction, hypoxia, and arousal during sleep impart significant sympathetic nervous system hyper-activation and hypertension which with hypoxaemia combine to increase the risk of ventricular arrhythmias. In addition the highly negative intra-thoracic pressure swings characteristic of increased ventilatory effort acting against a closed airway lead to worsened left ventricular after-load due to an increase in the transmural left ventricular pressure gradient. With an increasing frequency these episodes, cumulatively adversely affect the heart and contribute to the progression of HF including an increased risk for recurrent HF hospitalizations, ventricular arrhythmias and mortality.[6]

Identifying heart failure patients with OSA

Given the pathophysiological and prognostic significance of OSA in patients with HF, and the overlap in the risk factors for these two conditions clinicians should be aware of the possibility of OSA affecting their HF patients. It is recommended to consider the possibility of OSA whenever a HF patient complains of sleep related symptoms, reports worsened snoring or day-time sleepiness or is admitted for decompensation or more detailed assessment. Questioning the sleep partner of a patient is also highly valuable in identifying OSA patients. Additional signs and symptoms consistent with the presence of OSA include unusual daytime sleepiness, disturbed nocturnal breathing, disrupted sleep, nocturia, morning headaches, and diminished concentration and memory.[7]

OSA has traditionally been diagnosed by formal polysomnography (PSG), during an overnight sleep study in a sleep laboratory. The recent introduction of portable monitors offers an easier route to assess HF patients for the likelihood of OSA. Based on current guidelines, the PSG is diagnostic for OSA if respiratory monitoring demonstrates at least five obstructive hypoxaemic episodes per hour of sleep (or more than 15 in the absence of sleep related symptoms) and this frequency is defined as the apnoea-hypopnoea index (AHI).[8]

Treatment options for OSA

The mainstay of treatment for OSA is a positive airway pressure mask which can be used in mild moderate and severe OSA.[8] The need for therapy should be discussed with the patient and if the AHI is above 15/hr then treatment is indicated to reduce this to below 15. This is a consensus recommendation and no adequately powered clinical trials have shown this improves either mortality or the risk of disease progression. Compliance with mask therapy is limited and the need for on-going therapy and the willingness of a patient to continue may depend on whether there is a noticeable improvement in sleep related or daytime sleepiness symptoms induced by therapy. There are currently three primary types of these therapies: continuous positive airway pressure (CPAP), bi-level positive airway pressure (BiPAP) in which pressure levels decrease during exhalation, and BiPAP-adaptive servoventilation (ASV) in which the two pressures change due to sensors in the device.[9] The adverse effects of ASV in HFrEF patients with predominantly central sleep apnoea mean that this therapy should be reserved only for those with predominant OSA-type sleep apnoea (see chapter on CSA). Mask based therapy should be combined with life-style changes such as weight loss in the obese, regular exercise and the avoidance of alcohol and other sedatives prior to retiring for the night. Positioning the sleeping patient head-up can also help. Custom-made oral appliances that push the mandible forward or specially designed mouth guards can assist to a limited extent. Upper airway reconstructive surgery is occasionally used in severe cases unresponsive to or intolerant of mask therapy.

References

1. Jilek C, Krenn M, Sebah D, et al. Prognostic impact of sleep disordered breathing and its treatment in heart failure: an observational study. Eur J Heart Fail. 13: 68–75, 2011.
2. Khayat R, Jarjoura D, Porter K, et al. Sleep disordered breathing and post-discharge mortality in patients with acute heart failure. Eur Heart J. 36: 1463–69, 2015.
3. Coats AJ, Shewan LG. Measuring therapeutic efficacy in the treatment of central sleep apnoea in patients with heart failure. Int J Cardiol. 2016 Mar; 206 Suppl: S16–21. doi:10.1016/j.ijcard.2016.02.123.
4. Javaheri S: A mechanism of central sleep apnea in patients with heart failure. N Engl J Med. 341: 949–54, 1999.
5. Khoo MC, Kronauer RE, Strohl KP, et al. Factors inducing periodic breathing in humans: a general model. J Appl Physiol. 53: 644–59, 1982.
6. Bitter T, Westerheide N, Prinz C, et al. Cheyne-Stokes respiration and obstructive sleep apnoea are independent risk factors for malignant ventricular arrhythmias requiring appropriate cardioverter-defibrillator therapies in patients with congestive heart failure. Eur Heart J. 32: 61–74, 2011.
7. Somers VK, White DP, Amin R, et al. Sleep apnea and cardiovascular disease: an American Heart Association/American College of Cardiology Foundation scientific statement from the American Heart Association Council for High Blood Pressure Research Professional Education Committee, Council on Clinical Cardiology, Stroke Council, and Council on Cardiovascular Nursing. Circulation. 118: 1080–1111, 2008.

8. Epstein LJ, Kristo D, Strollo PJ Jr, et al. Adult Obstructive Sleep Apnea Task Force of the American Academy of Sleep Medicine. Clinical guideline for the evaluation, management and long-term care of obstructive sleep apnea in adults. J Clin Sleep Med. 2009 Jun 15; 5(3): 263–76.
9. El Shayeb M, Topfer LA, Stafinski T, et al. Diagnostic accuracy of level 3 portable sleep tests versus level 1 polysomnography for sleep-disordered breathing: a systematic review and meta-analysis. CMAJ. 186: E25–E51, 2014.

20

The management of co-morbidities in patients with heart failure – central sleep apnoea

Background

Despite many therapeutic advances, heart failure (HF) remains challenging to treat and continues to be associated with high rates of morbidity and mortality. There is an ongoing need to identify co-morbidities that either contribute to the progression of heart failure or limit the therapeutic response to treatment. One area under active investigation is the treatment of central sleep apnoea (CSA). CSA has consistently been shown to be associated with a worse prognosis in HF patients.[1–6] Thus, understanding how to diagnose and treat CSA is of paramount importance to the HF clinician.

CSA is a chronic respiratory disorder characterized by fluctuations in central, brainstem-driven respiratory drive that results in the cessation of respiratory muscle activity and airflow during sleep.[7] CSA is a common finding in HF, occurring in up to 40% of patients, and is seen in both HF with reduced ejection fraction and HF with preserved ejection fraction.[8–14] CSA in patients with HF is usually in the form of Cheyne-Stokes respiration[15–18] which is characterized by cycles of deep, rapid, crescendo-decrescendo breathing (hyperpnoea) followed by a period of slower, shallower breathing (hypopnoea) or no breathing at all (apnoea). The mechanism underlying the development of CSA in HF is respiratory control system instability due to oscillation of the arterial blood carbon dioxide level ($PaCO_2$) above and below the central threshold of ventilation termed the apnoeic threshold.[19–21] Multiple factors appear to contribute to respiratory control system instability and predispose HF patients to fluctuations in the $PaCO_2$, including lung congestion, elevation in sympathetic activation and reduced cardiac output leading to prolonged circulation time.[22–28] Often these factors lead to hyperventilation which drives the $PaCO_2$ below the apnoeic threshold, the brainstem-driven respiratory drive is supressed, and cessation of respiratory muscle activity and airflow (i.e., CSA) ensues. Resumption of breathing after an apnoeic episode does not occur until the chemical stimuli accumulate to relatively hypercapnic levels leading to a period of rapid breathing (hyperpnea) and triggering the next apnoeic event.

Pathophysiology

Each CSA cycle of apnea and hyperpnoea is associated with significant pauses in breathing or shallow breathing, with consequent hypoxia and arousals that cause severe disruption to the architecture of sleep and a surge in sympathetic

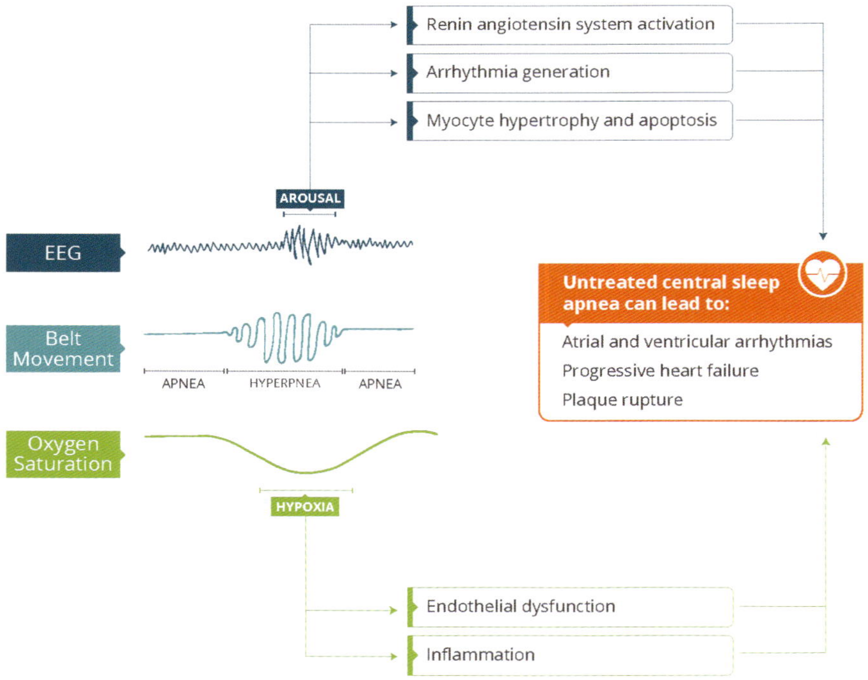

FIGURE 20.1 The pathophysiological consequences of CSA in heart failure

activity (Figure 20.1). Repeated cycles of apnoea, hypoxia, and arousal during sleep impart significant cardiovascular insults such as additional sympathetic nervous system activation, acute pulmonary and systemic hypertension, plaque rupture and arrhythmias.[1,29–31] As the cycles continue, these insults continue to adversely affect the heart and contribute to the downward cycle of HF including an increased risk for recurrent HF hospitalizations, ventricular arrhythmias and mortality (Figure 20.1).[3,6]

Identifying heart failure patients with CSA

Given the pathophysiological and prognostic significance of CSA in patients with HF, clinicians must maintain a high suspicion for CSA in HF patients. Additionally, patients should be evaluated for the presence of CSA when admitted to the hospital with acute decompensated HF, since signs of CSA such as shortness of breath at night often emerge with worsening HF. HF patients commonly have CSA risk factors including male gender, higher New York Heart Association class, lower left ventricular ejection fraction, waking hypocapnia, presence of atrial fibrillation, higher brain natriuretic peptide (BNP) levels, and frequent nocturnal ventricular arrhythmias.[8,10] Symptoms for CSA are more difficult to assess in patients with HF as many of the symptoms overlap with symptoms of HF such as fatigue or gasping at night. Additional signs and symptoms consistent with the presence of CSA include unusual daytime or night-time breathing patterns, disrupted sleep, nocturia, morning headaches, and diminished concentration and memory.[32] If possible, the patient's sleep partner should also be questioned about the patient's sleep habits, especially regarding episodes of apnoea, frequent arousals, or changes in behaviour or mood, which might signal the presence of CSA.

CSA traditionally has been diagnosed through polysomnography (PSG), or the overnight sleep study, which is performed in a sleep laboratory with a sleep technician in attendance. Based on current guidelines, the PSG is diagnostic for CSA if respiratory monitoring demonstrates at least three consecutive cycles of crescendo-decrescendo change in breathing amplitude and one or both of the following: 1) five or more central sleep apnoeas or hypopnoeas per sleep hour and/or 2) cyclical crescendo-decrescendo breathing $\geq$ 10 consecutive minutes.[33] CSA severity commonly is described by the apnoea-hypopnoea index (AHI), defined as the number of apnoea and hypopnoea events per hour of sleep[7] with an AHI $>$ 15 events/hour indicating moderate to severe CSA. While patients may have both CSA and OSA, the predominant form typically classifies the disorder.

While many patients go to the sleep laboratory for diagnosis, portable sleep monitors are designed to be used in an unattended, home-based setting. A number of different types of portable monitors are commercially available, with each device differing in the number and type of sleep-related variables they monitor. Level 3 portable monitors, which record at least 3 channels of data (e.g., oximetry, airflow, respiratory effort), have been shown to offer accurate diagnostic performance in HF patients and can distinguish obstructive from central events based on belt movement.[34] It is important for the clinician, however, to account for possible underestimation of the number of apnea events/hour with portable monitors as they are not able to monitor sleeping time.

Treatment options for CSA

Optimum treatment for HF patients with CSA has been limited. Current treatment options for CSA include medications, oxygen, positive airway pressure and neurostimulation of the phrenic nerve.[35] While a number of medications have been studied in small trials with acetazolamide and theophylline demonstrating some improvement in randomized trials, none are currently recommended due to lack of larger and longer term trials.[36] Oxygen has been used and improves symptoms in some studies, but no long term randomized trials have been completed.[36] Until recently, due the diagnosis of CSA primarily occurring in the sleep lab, positive airway pressure therapies historically used for the treatment of OSA were tested in the treatment of CSA. A very different approach using neurostimulation to stimulate the phrenic nerve and move the diaphragm to restore normal breathing has been developed.

Positive airway pressure therapies were initially utilized to open closed airways in patients with obstructive sleep apnoea. There are currently three primary types of these therapies: continuous positive airway pressure (CPAP), bi-level positive airway pressure (BiPAP) in which pressure levels decrease during exhalation, and BiPAP-adaptive servoventilation (ASV) in which the two pressures change due to sensors in the device.[37] The use of CPAP to treat CSA was studied in a large randomized, controlled trial, the Canadian Positive Airway Pressure Study (CANPAP). This trial was stopped early due to slow enrollment and safety concerns as the treatment group initially had a higher mortality than the treatment group.[38] However, over time, no difference in morbidity or mortality was seen. CPAP did improve the number of events per hour (40 to 19) and ejection fraction, but compliance with the therapy was low with an average use of 3.6 hours/night.

A newer form of positive airway pressure therapy, ASV, was designed specifically for the heart failure patient. It was expected that ASV would be able to deliver lower airway pressure to patients and adjust automatically to increase or lower pressure to maintain airflow. A large randomized study, the SERVE-HF trial, demonstrated that the AHI was greatly reduced while the patient wore the device. However, the trial also showed a surprising increase in both overall and cardiovascular mortality. While there is debate on the cause of the increased mortality, the pressure delivered was quite elevated in some patients and compliance remained an issue with patients utilizing therapy 3.2 hours/night.[39] Based on this data, ASV is now a Class III contraindication in the HF guidelines for patients with an ejection fraction less than 45%.

A novel physiologic approach to the treatment of CSA is now available using transvenous stimulation of the phrenic nerve. This system, the **rem**edē® System, was developed to physiologically address the treatment of CSA. As there is a delay in the signal from the brain to the phrenic nerve to stimulate the diaphragm in CSA, this system stimulates the phrenic nerve to prevent the apnoea or shallow breathing and is designed to normalize the breathing pattern.[40] Clinical data from the randomized controlled clinical trial was presented at the ESC-HFA meeting in May 2016. The trial met its primary endpoint; a greater proportion of patients in the treatment group having a ≥ 50% reduction in AHI compared to the control group at 6 months. In addition, pre-specified tested improvements in both respiratory metrics (AHI, central apneas, oxygenation, arousals and % of time in REM sleep) and in patient reported outcomes (Patient Global Assessment and Epworth Sleepiness Scale) were demonstrated. There were no safety concerns with 91% freedom from device related serious adverse events. While not powered, it was encouraging that no difference in either all-cause or cardiovascular mortality was noted. It is possible that a stronger recommendation for this therapeutic approach could have been included in recent guidelines had the data been available earlier.[41]

The future of CSA therapy

Central sleep apnoea is of paramount importance to the HF clinician. Without treatment, HF patients continue to be at risk for the devastating consequences of CSA. Prognosis is very poor with studies consistently demonstrating poor outcomes among HF patients with CSA. Over the course of the night, each discrete event contributes to increased nor-epinephrine levels and hypoxia which are associated with progressive heart failure and arrhythmias. Initial therapeutic options utilized therapies which were developed for obstructive sleep apnoea with limited success or even harm. ASV is now contraindicated in HF patients with an EF < 45% leaving only 2 potential treatment options: CPAP and transvenous phrenic nerve stimulation. Data from the recently presented (post ESC guidelines) trial on transvenous phrenic nerve stimulation demonstrated efficacy without the need for patient compliance or any safety concerns. It is expected that additional studies in CSA will continue to demonstrate the full impact of treating this important co-morbidity on patients with HF.

References

1. Lanfranchi PA, Braghiroli A, Bosimini E, et al. Prognostic value of nocturnal Cheyne-Stokes respiration in chronic heart failure. Circulation. 99: 1435–40, 1999.
2. Hanly PJ, Zuberi-Khokhar NS: Increased mortality associated with Cheyne-Stokes respiration in patients with congestive heart failure. Am J Resp Crit Care Med. 153: 272–6, 1996.
3. Javaheri S, Shukla R, Zeigler H, Wexler L: Central sleep apnea, right ventricular dysfunction and low diastolic blood pressure are predictors of mortality in systolic heart failure. J Am Coll Cardiol. 49: 2028–34, 2007.
4. Jilek C, Krenn M, Sebah D, et al. Prognostic impact of sleep disordered breathing and its treatment in heart failure: an observational study. Eur J Heart Fail. 13: 68–75, 2011.
5. Khayat R, Abraham W, Patt B, et al. Central sleep apnea is a predictor of cardiac readmission in hospitalized patients with systolic heart failure. J Cardiac Fail. 18: 534–40, 2012.
6. Khayat R, Jarjoura D, Porter K, et al. Sleep disordered breathing and post-discharge mortality in patients with acute heart failure. Eur Heart J. 36: 1463–69, 2015.
7. American Academy of Sleep Medicine. International classification of sleep disorders: diagnostic and coding manual. 2nd ed. Westchester, IL, 2005.
8. Oldenburg O, Lamp B, Faber L, et al. Sleep disordered breathing in patients with symptomatic heart failure: a contemporary study of prevalence in and characteristics of 700 patients. Eur J Heart Fail. 9: 251–7, 2007.
9. Javaheri S: Sleep disorders in systolic heart failure: a prospective study of 100 male patients. The final report. Int J Cardiol. 106: 21–8, 2006.
10. Sin DD, Fitzgerald F, Parker JD, et al. Risk factors for central and obstructive sleep apnea in 450 men and women with congestive heart failure. Am J Respir Crit Care Med. 160: 1101–6, 1999.
11. MacDonald M, Fang J, Pittman SD, et al. The current prevalence of sleep disordered breathing in congestive heart failure patients treated with beta-blockers. J Clin Sleep Med. 4: 38–42, 2008.
12. Chan J, Sanderson J, Chan W, et al. Prevalence of sleep-disordered breathing in diastolic heart failure. Chest. 111: 1488–93, 1999.
13. Herrscher TE, Akre H, Øverland B, et al. High prevalence of sleep apnea in heart failure outpatients: even in patients with preserved systolic function. J Card Fail. 17: 420–5, 2011.
14. Bitter T, Faber L, Hering D, et al. Sleep-disordered breathing in heart failure with normal left ventricular ejection fraction. Eur J Heart Fail. 11: 602–8, 2009.
15. Ward M: Periodic respiration. A short historical note. Ann R Coll Surg Engl. 52: 330–4, 1973.

16. Allen R, Truk JL, Muricy R: The Case Books of John Hunter, FRS. New York, Parthenon 1993.
17. Cheyne J: A case of apoplexy, in which the fleshy part of the heart was converted into fat. Dublin Hospital Reports and Communications. 2: 216–23, 1818.
18. Stokes W: Observations on some cases of permanently slow pulse. Dublin Quarterly Journal of Medical Sciences 2: 73–85, 1846.
19. Naughton M, Benard D, Tam A, et al. Role of hyperventilation in the pathogenesis of central sleep apneas in patients with congestive heart failure. Am Rev Respir Dis. 148: 330–8, 1993.
20. Hanly P, Zuberi N, Gray R: Pathogenesis of Cheyne-Stokes respiration in patients with congestive heart failure: relationship to arterial PCO2. Chest 104: 1079–84, 1993.
21. Dempsey JA: Crossing the apnoeic threshold: causes and consequences. Exp Physiol 90: 13–24, 2005.
22. Yu J, Zhang JF, Fletcher EC: Stimulation of breathing by activation of pulmonary peripheral afferents in rabbits. J Appl Physiol. 85: 1485–92, 1998.
23. Solin P, Bergin P, Richardson M: Influence of pulmonary capillary wedge pressure on central apnea in heart failure. Circulation. 99: 1574–9, 1999.
24. Lorenzi-Filho G, Azevedo ER, Parker JD, et al. Relationship of carbon dioxide tension in arterial blood to pulmonary wedge pressure in heart failure. Eur Respir J. 19: 37–40, 2002.
25. Javaheri S: A mechanism of central sleep apnea in patients with heart failure. N Engl J Med. 341: 949–54, 1999.
26. Solin P, Roebuck T, Johns DP, et al. Peripheral and central ventilatory responses in central sleep apnea with and without congestive heart failure. Am J Respir Crit Care Med. 162: 2194–200, 2000.
27. Khoo MC, Kronauer RE, Strohl KP, et al. Factors inducing periodic breathing in humans: a general model. J Appl Physiol. 53: 644–59, 1982.
28. Hall MJ, Xie A, Rutherford R, et al. Cycle length of periodic breathing in patients with and without heart failure. Am J Respir Crit Care Med. 154: 376–81, 1996.
29. Javaheri S, Dempsey JA: Central sleep apnea. Compr Physiol. 3: 141–63, 2013.
30. Naughton MT, Benard DC, Liu PP, et al. Effects of nasal CPAP on sympathetic activity in patients with heart failure and central sleep apnea. Am J Respir Crit Care Med. 152: 473–9, 1995.
31. Bitter T, Westerheide N, Prinz C, et al. Cheyne-Stokes respiration and obstructive sleep apnoea are independent risk factors for malignant ventricular arrhythmias requiring appropriate cardioverter-defibrillator therapies in patients with congestive heart failure. Eur Heart J. 32: 61–74, 2011.
32. Somers VK, White DP, Amin R, et al. Sleep apnea and cardiovascular disease: an American Heart Association/American College of Cardiology Foundation scientific statement from the American Heart Association Council for High Blood Pressure Research Professional Education Committee, Council on Clinical Cardiology, Stroke Council, and Council on Cardiovascular Nursing. Circulation. 118: 1080–1111, 2008.
33. Sleep-related breathing disorders in adults: recommendations for syndrome definition and measurement techniques in clinical research. The report of an American Academy of Sleep Medicine Task Force. Sleep. 22: 667–89, 1999.

34. El Shayeb M, Topfer LA, Stafinski T, et al. Diagnostic accuracy of level 3 portable sleep tests versus level 1 polysomnography for sleep-disordered breathing: a systematic review and meta-analysis. CMAJ. 186: E25–E51, 2014.
35. Costanzo MR, Khayat R, Ponikowski P et al. Mechanisms and clinical consequences of untreated central sleep apnea in heart failure. J Am Coll Cardiol 2015; 65: 72–84.
36. Aurora RN; Chowdhuri S; Ramar K; Bista SR; Casey KR; Lamm CI; Kristo DA; Mallea JM; Rowley JA; Zak RS; Tracy SL. The treatment of central sleep apnea syndromes in adults: practice parameters with an evidence-based literature review and meta-analyses. SLEEP 2012; 35(1): 17–40.
37. Khayat RN; Abraham WT. Current treatment approaches and trials in central sleep apnea. Int J Cardiol 2016; 206: S22–S27.
38. Bradley TD, Logan AG, Kimoff RJ et al. Continuous positive airway pressure for central sleep apnea and heart failure. N Engl J Med 2005; 353: 2025–33.
39. Cowie MR, Wegscheider K, Teschler H. Adaptive Servo-Ventilation for Central Sleep Apnea in Heart Failure. N Engl J Med 2016; 374: 690–1.
40. Abraham WT, Jagielski D, Oldenburg O, Augostini R, Krueger S, Kolodziej A, Gutleben KJ, Khayat R, Merliss A, Harsch MR, Holcomb RG, Javaheri S, Ponikowski P on behalf of the remedē® Pilot Study Investigators. Phrenic Nerve Stimulation for the Treatment of Central Sleep Apnea. JCHF 2015; 5: 360–369.
41. Costanzo MR, Ponikowski P, Augostini R, Goldberg L, Holcomb R, Javaheri S, Kao A, Oldenburg O, Stellbrink C, Abraham WT, for the remed System Pivotal Trial Study Group. Pivotal trial of transvenous phrenic nerve stimulation for central sleep apnea. Late-breaking clinical trials ESC-HFA. May 2016.

21

The management of co-morbidities in patients with heart failure – potassium balance

Background

Both hypokalaemia and hyperkalaemia are common in HF patients. They are each associated both with HF and with the many drugs used for HF. They are important as they both can aggravate ventricular arrhythmias, both can cause symptoms in HF patients and in the case of hyperkalaemia in particular, are a common reason not to prescribe or reduce the dose of or even cease use of effective medication with life-prolonging benefits in HFrEF, including ACEI's and MRA's.

Potassium control

90% of the body's stores of potassium (K^+) are held intracellularly. What is measured in plasma represents less than 1% of total body K^+. Serum potassium is normally regulated within a narrow range of 3.5 to 5.0 mmol/L, despite large variation in intake through food and drinks. Homeostasis is maintained both by control of the renal excretion and loss from the gut, and by regulating movements of K^+ between intracellular and extracellular compartments. Excretion in HF is abnormal because of the use of diuretics (loop and thiazides increase excretion) and because of impaired renal blood flow and GFR. Aldosterone elevation increases potassium loss and internal shifts of K^+ are under the influence of insulin and catecholamines, both of which mechanisms are altered in HF. Lastly ACEI's, ARB's and MRA's all increase K^+ levels in the serum.

Renal K^+ excretion is mediated by aldosterone and by GFR.[1] K^+ is filtered by the glomerulus, and partially reabsorbed in the proximal tubule, paralleling sodium and water exchange. This absorption in the proximal part of the nephron passively follows that of Na+ and water, whereas reabsorption in the thick ascending limb of the loop of Henle is mediated by a Na/K/Cl carrier (NKCC2). K^+ is later secreted by the connecting segment, the cortical and outer medullary collecting tubule, and the collecting duct via luminal potassium channels. and the activity of this secretion largely determines the degree of urinary K^+ loss through the kidney, although reabsorption through the intercalated cells in the cortical and outer medullary collecting tubules via an active ATPase pump can affect K^+ loss.

Hypokalaemia

Hypokalaemia when usually defined as a serum potassium concentration below 3.5 mmol/L is found in about 20% of hospitalized patients, most frequently in HF and multi-organ failure patients. Hypokalaemia can result from alterations in both long term (largely renal) or short term (transcellular shifts) or by excessive potassium losses from the gut, such as in severe diarrhoea. Transcellular shifts can occur in response to a surge in catecholamines or by acid-base disturbances. Loop or thiazide diuretic use and hyper-aldosteronism both worsen renal potassium losses in CHF.

Hypokalaemia is frequently detected only by routine blood testing. Symptoms to make one suspicious may include muscle weakness, constipation, or worsening ectopy or higher grade arrhythmias. In CHF, even mild hypokalaemia may worsen ventricular arrhythmias. Severe hypokalaemia can rarely cause myopathy and paralysis with the risk of respiratory arrest at levels <2.0 mmol/L.

The treatment of mild hypokalaemia detected routinely can involve recommending high potassium foods or prescribing potassium supplements, although these should be reviewed regularly because of the risk of hyperkalaemia in these patients. Intravenous potassium administration is rarely indicated because of the risk of overshoot hyperkalaemia, except for very difficult to control arrhythmias in which case continuous monitoring, with no more than 20 mmol/hr K^+administered, and regular reassessment of the serum potassium level after every 60 mmol is given. Concomitant hypomagnesaemia may need to be corrected at the same time effective to correct the hypokalaemia fully.

Hyperkalaemia

Hyperkalemia is defined as a serum potassium concentration higher than 5.0 mmol/L. Pseudohyperkalemia can occur with haemolysis, so repeat testing taking blood without a tourniquet is recommended before aggressive treatment is started if this is suspected.

Hyperkalaemia occurs in 1% to 10% of all hospitalized patients with a noticeable increase in HF.[2,3] after the widespread uptake of MRA's for HF after the results of the RALES study. Most hyperkalaemia is caused by impaired potassium excretion from renal insufficiency. Drugs such ACEI's, ARB's MRA's and potassium-sparing diuretics (e.g., spironolactone, triamterene, sometimes used as adjunct diuretics in resistant oedema, or to assist in preventing hypokalaemia) will increase the risk of hyperkalaemia. Nonsteroidal anti-inflammatory drugs (NSAIDs) and heparin can also impair the excretion of K^+.

Hyperkalaemia is frequently detected by routine blood testing. Symptoms and signs to make one suspicious include muscle weakness, cardiac conduction disturbances, "tented" T waves, QRS widening, and bradycardia, however these ECG changes are not closely related to the level of serum potassium. The toxic effects of hyperkalaemia can be enhanced by hypocalcaemia, hyponatraemia and acidosis.[4] Severe severe acute hyperkalaemia (>6 mol/l) can lead to cardiac arrest and death,[5] with a mortality rates of up to 30% in severe uncorrected hyperkalaemia.[6]

The management of severe acute hyperkalaemia (>6 mol/l) may require short-term cessation of potassium retaining agents and inhibitors of the RAAS, but this should be minimized and RAAS inhibitors should be carefully reintroduced as soon as possible whilst monitoring potassium levels. Other emergency treatments include intravenous insulin and glucose, nebulized or inhaled beta-2–receptor agonists and calcium gluconate salts. Haemodialysis may be required in severe prolonged hyperkalaemia. A Cochrane review found no trial evidence of major outcome benefit for any emergency hyperkalaemia therapy with the best efficacy when medical (as opposed to dialysis) potassium lowering is required was for beta agonists and intravenous insulin-and-glucose.[7] The safety of neither therapy has been established specifically in the HF population. In view of their risks beta agonists are usually avoided in HF.

For chronic management of the risk of hyperkalaemia gut-active potassium binding agents have been shown to lower serum potassium including in HF patients and trial evidence to assess their long term safety and benefit in HF would be valuable. For patients at risk of serious hyperkalaemia chronically, sodium polystyrene sulfonate (an ion-exchange resin that binds potassium in the colon) has been used but it frequently causes gastrointestinal disturbance as well as increasing the risk of sodium loading, hypomagnesaemia, hypocalcaemia, and colonic necrosis.

One frequently under-recognised risk of high potassium levels (even if only intermittent) is that evidence-based, life-saving medications may be under-dosed or stopped altogether. This could put patients at increased risk and could in the end be an increased burden to health care costs due to increased re-hospitalisation rates for HF. Therefore there is an important unmet need for novel therapeutic options for the long-term management of patients with, and at risk for, hyperkalaemia. Newer potassium binders for the treatment of hyperkalaemia have recently been approved.[8] Patiromer is a cation exchange polymer that exchanges calcium for potassium in the GI tract. It decreases serum potassium, and protects against episodes of recurrent hyperkalaemia. In the OPAL-HK trial this has been shown to reduce the need discontinuation of RAAS inhibitors[9] an outcome likely to be of significant clinical benefit in HF patients. In this trial in CKD patients (42% also with heart failure) with baseline potassium levels of 5.1–6.5 mmol/l treated initially with open label patiromer were then randomised to double blind continuation of patiromer or withdrawal (control) over 8 weeks. A recurrence of hyperkalaemia (potassium level, ≥5.5 mmol/l) occurred in only 15% of patiromer treated patients compared to 60% in control patients up to 8 weeks ($p<0.001$). All the patients were receiving at least one RAAS inhibitor at baseline and at the end of the randomized withdrawal phase, 44% in the placebo group as compared with 94% in the patiromer group were still receiving RAAS inhibitors. If this difference could be maintained long term there may well be significant survival benefits of using this agent long term HF patients at high risk of hyperkalaemia if indeed effective doses of ACEI's and MRA's can be maintained significantly more frequently by such a strategy.

In a pre-specified analysis of HF patients in OPAL-HK 142 patients (42% of the overall trial) the change in serum K^+ from baseline to week 4 was -1.06 ± 0.05 mEq/L and 76% of patients achieved serum K^+ levels of 3.8 mEq/L to <5.1 mEq/L. In the randomized withdrawal phase, the median increase in serum K^+ from baseline of that phase was greater with placebo ($n = 22$) than patiromer ($n = 27$) ($P < 0.001$) and recurrent hyperkalaemia (serum K+, ≥5.5 mEq/L) occurred in 52% on placebo and 8% on patiromer ($P < 0.001$), confirmer similar efficacy and safety in HF patients.

Two other trials (PEARL-HF and AMETHYST-DN) examined the safety and efficacy of patiromer in patients with hyperkalemia or at risk for hyperkalaemia and receiving RAAS inhibitors. The PEARL-HF study increased the proportion of patients able to titrate their spironolactone dose from 25 mg/day to 50 mg/day in patients with a history of hyperkalemia or an eGFR of <60 mL/

min. The AMETHYST-DN study demonstrated that patiromer maintained mean serum potassium ≤5.0 mEq/L for up to 1 year with a low rate of hypokalemia.[10] The increasing evidence suggest agents such as patiromer may be safe and effective agents to be used long-term in high-risk patients with HF to allow them to take doses of RAAS inhibitors in particular which they otherwise may not be able to take. This would allow them to continue to receive the mortality morbidity benefits these treatments confer.

References

1. Gennari FJ, Segal AS: Hyperkalemia: An adaptive response in chronic renal insufficiency. Kidney Int. 2002; 62: 1–9.
2. Sarafidis PA, Blacklock R, Wood E, et al. Prevalence and factors associated with hyperkalemia in predialysis patients followed in a low-clearance clinic, Clin J Am Soc Nephrol. 2012; 7: 1234–41.
3. Desai AS, Hyperkalemia in patients with heart failure: incidence, prevalence, and management, Curr Heart Fail Rep. 2009; 6: 272–80.
4. Charytan D, Goldfarb DS: Indications for hospitalization of patients with hyperkalemia. Arch Intern Med. 2000; 160: 1605–1611.
5. Korgaonkar S, Tilea A, Gillespie BW, et al. Serum potassium and outcomes in CKD: insights from the RRI-CKD cohort study, Clin J Am Soc Nephrol. 2010; 5: 762–9.
6. An JN, Lee JP, Jeon HJ, et al. Severe hyperkalemia requiring hospitalization: predictors of mortality, Crit Care. 2012; 16: R225.
7. Mahoney BA, Smith WAD, Lo D, Tsoi K, Tonelli M, Clase C. Emergency interventions for hyperkalaemia. Cochrane Database of Systematic Reviews 2005, Issue 2. Art. No.: CD003235. doi:10.1002/14651858.CD003235.pub2.
8. FDA, FDA approves new drug to treat hyperkalemia. http://www.fda.gov/NewsEvents/Newsroom/PressAnnouncements/ucm468546.htm
9. Weir MR, Bakris GL, Bushinsky DA, et al. Patiromer in patients with kidney disease and hyperkalemia receiving RAAS inhibitors. N Engl J Med. 2015; 372: 211–21.
10. Montaperto, Ann G; Gandhi, Mona A; Gashlin, Lauren Z; Symoniak, Melanie R Patiromer: a clinical review. 2016; 32: 155–64. doi:10.1185/03007995.2015.1106935

22

The management of co-morbidities in patients with heart failure – iron deficiency

Background

Co-morbidities have been recognised as playing a crucial role in the progress of the older patient with HF in particular. The 2016 ESC/HFA HF guidelines stress the significance of co-morbidities more than any previous guidelines have.[1] Figure 22.1 lists the reasons for the importance of directing attention to co-morbidities frequent in the HF patient. Iron deficiency is one such co-morbidity, that has received very little attention until the last decade, as evidence has accumulated both for the significance of this co-morbidity and the emergence of safe effective therapies that appear to offer significant benefits to the HF population who suffer this co-morbidity.

Iron deficiency (defined as serum ferritin <100 m/L or ferritin between 100 and 299 mg/L with a transferrin saturation <20%) is common in HF, as it is with other chronic illnesses. When present it is associated with a more progressive course of HF, more hospitalisations, worse symptomatology and an impaired prognosis. It can also lead to anaemia (defined as a haemoglobin concentration <13 g/dL in men and <12 g/dL in women) and skeletal muscle dysfunction. It has been a distraction that iron deficiency can cause anaemia because attention has been directed to attempts to correct the anaemia itself, which is also common in HF patients, but transfusions and erythropoietic agents have not been shown to be beneficial in HF patients specially. If anaemia is present a cause should be sought such as the search for a bleeding diathesis or local site of blood loss, along with iron, folate and

1. interfere with the diagnostic process of HF (e.g. COPD as a potentially confounding cause of dyspnoea).[390,391]
2. aggravate HF symptoms and further impair quality of life.[391,392]
3. contribute to the burden of hospitalizations and mortality,[393] as the main cause of readmissions at 1 and 3 months.[394]
4. may affect the use of treatments for HF (e.g. renin–angiotensin system inhibitors contra-indicated in some patients with severe renal dysfunction or beta-blockers relatively contra-indicated in asthma).[395,396]
5. evidence base for HF treatment is more limited as co-morbidities were mostly an exclusion criterion in trials; efficacy and safety of interventions is therefore often lacking in the presence of co-morbidities.
6. drugs used to treat co-morbidities may cause worsening HF (e.g. NSAIDs given for arthritis, some anti-cancer drugs).[397]
7. interaction between drugs used to treat HF and those used to treat co-morbidities, resulting in lower efficacy, poorer safety, and the occurrence of side effects (e.g. beta-blockers for HFrEF and beta-agonists for COPD and asthma).[391,395,396]

FIGURE 22.1 Importance of co-morbidities in patients with HF. Numbers in the table refer to references in the ESC/HFA guidelines[1]

B12 deficiency. But it is iron deficiency in particular, rather than the anaemia it can cause which has been a success story in our attempts to find and correct a co-morbidity of importance for our HF patients. Anaemia is more frequent in women, the elderly, in the presence of kidney impairment and in acutely hsopitalised HF patients. In many patients no specific cause is found. When present there appears to be more marked myocardial remodeling, inflammation and volume overload.[2] Anaemia is associated with more symptoms, worse functional status, greater risk of HF hospitalization, and reduced survival. The 2016 guidelines warn that erythropoietin-stimulating agent darbepoetin alfa did not improve clinical outcomes in HFREF patients with mild-to-moderate anemia but led to an excess of thrombo-embolic events and is therefore not recommended.[1,3]

Significance of iron deficiency

Within a HF population iron deficiency (ID) is associated with a worse prognosis.[4] In a large cohort of CHF patients ID was identified in nearly 50%.[5] Although anaemic patients were more often iron deficient than those without anaemia, the difference was surprisingly small (61.2% vs 45.6%, $P < .001$). Other independent predictors of ID were worse symptoms, N-terminal

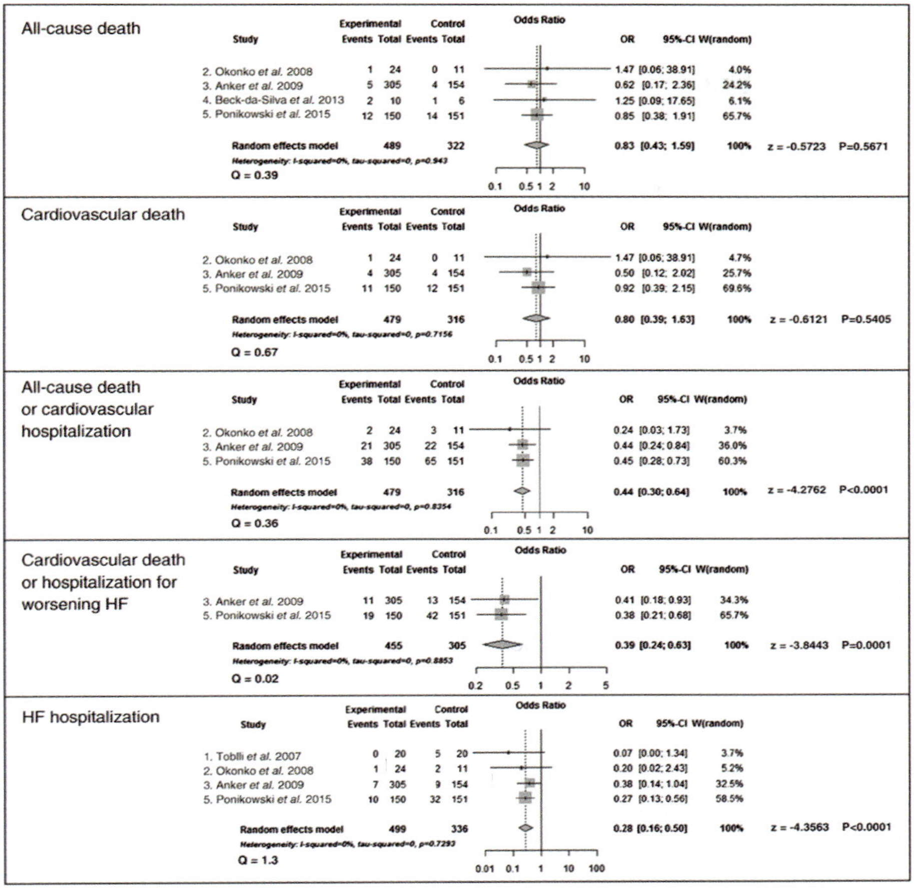

FIGURE 22.2 Effects of intravenous iron therapy in iron-deficient patients with systolic heart failure: a meta-analysis of randomized controlled trials.[15] Effects of intravenous iron therapy on outcomes in patients with systolic heart failure (HF) and iron deficiency. CI, confidence interval, HF, heart failure; OR, odds ratio.

pro-BNP and female gender. Functional ID is described as impaired mobilization of iron from iron stores which remain normal (such as is seen in the anaemia of chronic disorders). Hepcidin and soluble transferrin receptor (sTfR) are also of importance if HF as they regulate of iron homeostasis, usage and uptake. Circulating levels of hepcidin are regulated by iron stores, whereas sTfR levels reflect tissue iron demand increasing to facilitate intracellular iron transfer. Absolute ID (often with very low hepcidin levels) is the predominant form of ID seen in HF, both acute and chronic.

Iron has several crucial roles in the body; haemopoiesis, oxygen transport and storage, cardiac and skeletal muscle metabolism, and mitochondrial function.[7] Myocardial iron stores are alos important determinants of myocardial function. Transferrin receptor-1 (TfR1) mRNA expression is reduced in the failing heart.[8] and was impaired by aldosterone and norepinephrine. These interactions might suggest broader benefits for iron therapy in HF.

Treatment options for iron deficiency

Therapeutic I.V. iron has been studied in HF both with and without anaemia. Anaemia does not appear to be needed for the therapeutic benefit of IV Iron. I.V. ferric carboxymaltose (FMC) has been shown to improve self-reported patient global assessment and NYHA class (over six months). The FAIR-HF trial[9] enrolled 459 class II or III, HFrEF randomly assigned 2:1 to 200 mg of IV FCM or placebo. Self-reported patient global assessment and NYHA class were both significantly improved, regardless of anaemia status. 6-minute walk test and quality-of-life assessments were also improved, with similar rates of death, adverse events, and serious adverse events. The CONFIRM-HF trial[10] using IV FCM showed a significant improvement in functional capacity in HFrEF patients (6 minute CWT +33±11 m, p=0.002) over 52 weeks. The beneficial effect was consistent in all subgroups and there was an associated improvement in NYHA class, PGA, QoL, and Fatigue Scores with a significant reduction in the risk of hospitalizations for worsening HF [hazard ratio (95% confidence interval): 0.39 (0.19–0.82), P = 0.009]. The number of deaths (FCM: 12, placebo: 14 deaths) and the incidence of adverse events were comparable between both groups. Overall these studies show that iron-deficient HF patients treated with IV FCM over a 1-year period resulted in prolonged improved functional capacity, symptoms, and QoL and may be associated with risk reduction of hospitalization for worsening HF. A meta-analysis of IV FCM in HFrEF patients with iron deficiency showed reduced hospitalization rates and improved HF symptoms, exercise capacity and quality of life.[11] 5 (n=907) reporting the clinical impact of iron therapy in patients with HF with ID compared with no iron treatment were analysed. Iron therapy was seen to be associated with a significantly reduced rate of hospitalization for HF (odds ratio [OR], 0.28; 95% confidence interval [CI], 0.16–0.49), and although all-cause mortality was not significantly different (OR, 0.81; 95% CI, 0.42–1.57) in trended in the same direction. The incidence of hospitalization for HF and death was lowered in the iron supplementation group (OR, 0.47; 95% CI, 0.29–0.76) and there was no increase in adverse event risk. Three of these studies (including the 3 largest)[9,10,12] used IV FCM and two used IV Iron sucrose.[13,14] It is fair to conclude that the proven beneficial effects of IV Iron are only reliably established for IV FCM preparation at present and not other forms of IV iron or oral iron. There are insufficient trial data to show any benefit of oral iron therapy in HF, especially given the severely depleted iron stores in HF. A second meta-analysis consisting of an aggregate data meta-analysis (random effects model) of randomized controlled trials that evaluated the effects of i.v. iron therapy in iron-deficient patients with systolic HF showed that IV iron reduces the risk of the combined endpoint of all-cause death or cardiovascular hospitalization [odds ratio (OR) 0.44, 95% confidence interval (CI) 0.30–0.64, $P < 0.0001$], and the combined endpoint of cardiovascular death or hospitalization for worsening HF (OR 0.39, 95% CI 0.24–0.63, $P = 0.0001$), along with improved NYHA class, quality of life and Patient Global Assessment (PGA).[15] The effect of treating iron deficiency in HFpEF remains unproven, but it is under active study.

Conclusions

Based on the evidence reviewed in this chapter and especially the two recent meta-analyses the reason for a strong new recommendation in the 2016 ESC/HFA guidelines on HF management are made clear. For the first time this important co-morbidity is given a clear tabular recommendation, that of a class IIA, A recommendation that "Intravenous FCM should be considered in symptomatic patients with HFrEF and iron deficiency (serum ferritin <100 m/L or ferritin between 100 and 299 mg/L with a transferrin saturation <20%) in order to alleviate HF symptoms, and to improve exercise capacity and quality of life." Furthermore, they suggest screening HF patients for ID by measuring Ferritin and TSAT. Evidence that it may well improve major outcomes is tantalisingly close. The evidence is, however, strong enough to suggest that all HFrEF patients should be screened for iron deficiency and when found IV FCM should be a standard part of what the HF physician can offer to improve the lives of the patients with HFrEF.

References

1. Ponikowski P, Voors A, Anker S et al The Task Force for the diagnosis and treatment of acute and chronic heart failure of the European Society of Cardiology (ESC). 2016 ESC Guidelines for the diagnosis and treatment of acute and chronic heart failure. European Journal of Heart Failure. Published online 26 May 2016.
2. O'Meara, E; Rouleau JL; White, M; et al. Heart Failure With Anemia. Circ Heart Fail. 2014; 7: 773–781.

3. Swedberg, K, Young JB, Anand, IS, et al. Treatment of Anemia with Darbepoetin Alfa in Systolic Heart Failure N Engl J Med 2013; 368: 1210–1219.
4. Jankowska EA, Malyszko J, Ardehali H, Koc-Zorawska E, Banasiak W, von Haehling S, Macdougall IC, Weiss G, McMurray JJ, Anker SD, Gheorghiade M, Ponikowski P. Iron status in patients with chronic heart failure. Eur Heart J. 2013; 34: 827–34.
5. I.T. Klip, J. Comin-Colet, A.A. Voors, et al. Iron deficiency in chronic heart failure: an international pooled analysis. Am Heart J, 165 (2013), pp. 575–582. e3.
6. O'Meara E; de Denus S; Lepage S. Heart Failure, Iron Deficiency, and Supplementation: Where Do We Stand?. Canadian Journal of Cardiology. 32(2): 148–50, 2016 Feb.
7. E.A. Jankowska, S. von Haehling, S.D. Anker, I.C. Macdougall, P. Ponikowski. Iron deficiency and heart failure: diagnostic dilemmas and therapeutic perspectives Eur Heart J, 34 (2013), pp. 816–829.
8. M.T. Maeder, O. Khammy, C. dos Remedios, D.M. Kaye. Myocardial and systemic iron depletion in heart failure implications for anemia accompanying heart failure. J Am Coll Cardiol, 58 (2011), pp. 474–480.
9. Anker SD, Comin Colet J, Filippatos G, et al. Ferric carboxymaltose in patients with heart failure and iron deficiency. N Engl J Med 2009; 361: 2436–2448.
10. P. Ponikowski, D.J. van Veldhuisen, J. Comin-Colet, et al. Beneficial effects of long-term intravenous iron therapy with ferric carboxymaltose in patients with symptomatic heart failure and iron deficiency. Eur Heart J, 36 (2015), pp. 657–668.
11. C. Qian, B. Wei, J. Ding, H. Wu, Y. Wang. The efficacy and safety of iron supplementation in patients with heart failure and iron deficiency: a systematic review and meta-analysis. Can J Cardiol, 32 (2016), pp. 151–159.
12. G. Arutyunov, N. Bylova, A. Ivleva, Z. Kobalava. The safety of intravenous (IV) ferric carboxymaltose versus IV iron sucrose in patients with chronic heart failure (CHF) and chronic kidney disease (CKD) with iron deficiency (ID). Eur J Heart Fail Suppl, 8 (2009) Abstract 141.
13. D.O. Okonko, A. Grzeslo, T. Witkowski, et al. Effect of intravenous iron sucrose on exercise tolerance in anemic and nonanemic patients with symptomatic chronic heart failure and iron deficiency FERRIC-HF: a randomized, controlled, observer-blinded trial. J Am Coll Cardiol, 51 (2008), pp. 103–112.
14. J.E. Toblli, A. Lombrana, P. Duarte, F. Di Gennaro. Intravenous iron reduces NT-pro-brain natriuretic peptide in anemic patients with chronic heart failure and renal insufficiency. J Am Coll Cardiol, 50 (2007), pp. 1657–1665.
15. Effects of intravenous iron therapy in iron-deficient patients with systolic heart failure: a meta-analysis of randomized controlled trials. Jankowska EA, Tkaczyszyn M, Suchocki T, Drozd M, von Haehling S, Doehner W, Banasiak W, Filippatos G, Anker SD, Ponikowski P. Eur J Heart Fail. 2016 Jan 28. doi:10.1002/ejhf.473.